Praise for CANCER SELF-HELP GRₒ

"For anyone who ever considered starting a cancer support group, this book will give you the courage and guidance you need to make your dream a reality."
—*Susan Love, MD, author of* Dr. Susan Love's Breast Book *and Founder,* *www.susanlovemd.com*

"An exceptional book, well-organized and easy to read. The author provides useful advice on just about every aspect of creating and maintaining an effective group. This is a superb resource for those in any type of self-help group."
—*Joal Fisher, MD, Founder and Director, SupportWorks*

Cancer Self-Help Groups: A Guide

Pat Kelly

FIREFLY BOOKS

To my daughters – Kate and Kelly – for teaching me about compassion
to Hugh for teaching me about grace and grits, and
to the people in our workshops who create the communities of caring.

All royalties from the sale of this book will be donated to cancer self-help groups.

A Firefly Book

Published by Firefly Books (U.S.) Inc. 2000

First Printing

U.S. CATALOGING IN PUBLICATION DATA

Kelly, Pat
    Cancer self-help groups : a guide / Pat Kelly. 1st U.S. ed.
[176]p. : cm.   – (Your Personal Health)
Originally published: A Guide for Cancer Self-Help Groups: Leadership from the Heart, Toronto: Key Porter, 1999.
Includes bibliographical references and index.
Summary: Guide to establishing and leading cancer support groups.
ISBN 1-55209-478-2
1. Social networks. 2. Cancer – Patients – Services for. 3. Cancer – Societies, etc.
I. Title. II. Series.
362.19 / 6994   21   2000   CIP

Published in the United States in 2000 by
Firefly Books (U.S.) Inc.
P.O. Box 1338, Ellicott Station
Buffalo, New York, USA
14205

Published in Canada in 2000 by Key Porter Books Limited.

Electronic formatting: Peter Ross/Heidi Palfrey
Design: Counterpunch

Printed and bound in Canada

ACKNOWLEDGMENTS

In keeping with the spirit of self-help, this manual has been a cooperative effort on the part of a small group of committed people. The information in this manual has come from a variety of sources, including real-life experiences of people involved with cancer groups, existing self-help materials, published research on self-help/mutual aid. Wherever possible, we have indicated the original source of the materials used.

Our thanks and appreciation are offered to the following people who generously gave time and effort to help this manual become a reality:

Dr. Juanne Nancarrow Clarke, Professor of Medical Sociology, Wilfrid Laurier University, Waterloo, Ontario

Dr. Alistair Cunningham, Clinical Co-director, Wellspring Cancer Resource Centre, Princess Margaret Hospital, Toronto, Ontario

Maureen O'Connor, Founder, Wellwood Cancer Resource Centre, Hamilton, Ontario

Mridula Sood, Program Coordinator, Bayview Support Network, Toronto, Ontario

Dr. Simon Sutcliffe, Vice-president, British Columbia Cancer Agency, Vancouver, British Columbia

Joal Fisher, MD, Support Works, Charlotte, North Carolina

David Cella, Ph.D., Director, Center on Outcomes, Research, and Education

Linda Frame, The Susan G. Komen Breast Cancer Foundation

Beverley Rogers, Y-ME National Breast Cancer Organization

Crystal Walsh, The Susan G. Komen Breast Cancer Foundation

Ellie Lang, Indiana

Carol Forhan, California

Elaine Hill, Tennessee

Lorna Patrick, Washington, DC

Barbara Oliver, Connecticut

Betty Kaiser, Arizona

Catherine Traiforou, New York

Catalino Ramos, Chicago

CONTENTS

INTRODUCTION

In 2000, more than 1,221,800 new cases of cancer will be diagnosed in the United States.[1] Along with the diagnosis, people often experience feelings of fear and loneliness. Many people with cancer have found caring, support, and information from self-help groups for cancer patients and survivors, and have learned how to change the loneliness and fear of their diagnosis into a journey of hope and healing. A measure of the success of cancer self-help groups is their ever-increasing numbers. In the eighties, the United States had few cancer self-help groups. Today, there are thousands of established groups across the country.

> *The beauty of a support group is that you don't have to explain anything. Many people with cancer try to shield family and friends from what they're going through. Sometimes they hide how scared or angry they feel. In a support group, you don't have to protect anyone. They're there to support you.*

Creating and maintaining an effective group is not always easy. This manual – written by and for cancer patients, in collaboration with researchers and other experts – outlines some of the strategies cancer survivors have discovered and the skills they have developed to meet the challenges of forming and working with their own support groups.

The manual builds upon the lessons learned from cancer patients who have started groups and participated as group members, and their stories have been included to help illustrate points in the text.

THE PURPOSE OF THIS MANUAL

The purpose of this manual is to offer encouragement and ideas to:
- people who want to start a cancer self-help group;
- people who are members of an established group;
- people who are thinking about facilitating a group;
- people who are struggling with problems in cancer groups.

There are high expectations placed upon self-help groups to deliver services in a timely and effective manner – a task that requires an understanding of group skills. At the same time, groups need to be able to stay in touch with their simple, grass-roots nature. This manual uses the expertise of cancer patients, survivors, and researchers to teach the group skills that will be appropriate to the unique needs of people with cancer.

Right from the start, it is important to understand the basic nature of self-help work. Helping is not done *for* others. It is done *with* others, *for* ourselves, recognizing that helping others creates meaning in our own lives. Simply put, self-help is a way to help both ourselves and others by paying attention to the suffering caused by cancer. When we see our own fear reflected in the eyes of someone who has just been diagnosed, we remember how important it was for us not just to learn more about cancer and its treatments but also to find someone to talk to about it. When we see relief and hope begin to strengthen that person again, we are rewarded. That is the spirit of self-help: helping others helps us.

All of us are interdependent. Whether we realize it or not, each of us lives eternally in the red.

Martin Luther King, Jr.

Here are some initial "words of wisdom" for anyone who is starting or helping out with a cancer self-help group:

- Think "share" from the beginning and reach out to others who share your vision.
- Take risks and be forgiving of your own mistakes and those of others.
- Remember that the most important gift we can bring is the quality of our attention.

Last but not least, remember that there is no one *right* way to do this. This manual is intended to be a guide, not a book of rules. You are not expected to do everything the way it is described here. Take what you need and leave the rest. You can come back when and if you need something else.

We have tried to combine the "art" of living with cancer with the "science" of building effective groups to sketch a road map for a journey that we hope will enlighten you – both intellectually and spiritually.

The Self-help Spirit: Connecting as a Way of Healing[2]

Do not close your eyes before suffering. Find ways to be with those who are suffering. By such means, awaken yourself and others to the reality of suffering in the world.

Gautama Buddha

The group members we talked with for this manual most commonly described the terrible sense of loneliness, fear, and loss of control they felt when they were first diagnosed with cancer. Again and again, people talked about the need for information and the need to meet others living with cancer – because other cancer survivors[3] symbolize hope.

There is a special bond between people with cancer. One researcher[4] described it this way:

> There seemed to be a kind of connecting that did not require words and which occurred with a startling immediacy and intensity. This instant bonding was experienced as unique in the lives of many with whom we talked.

In all of the cancer self-help groups, survivors talked about the importance of belonging to a group where they didn't need to explain themselves – where everyone has a cancer story.

People with cancer who participate in groups use storytelling as a way to connect with others in an immediate and intimate way. Storytelling helps us to get through the loneliness and regain a sense of control.

> It was tremendous – that experience! I just remember walking in for the first time and being, you know, somewhat nervous, not knowing who was going to be at the meeting. But I remember driving home afterwards with my mom and just beaming because of walking into this room and meeting strangers and people I didn't know, but just to have this one common thing! Lauren, diagnosed with leukemia at age 17

Cancer survivors use a variety of stories to describe what it is like to have cancer. One story compares cancer to being a Vietnam War veteran.

When I returned from Vietnam I felt like the world was made up of two kinds of people: those who were in Vietnam and those who weren't. People who weren't couldn't understand me. People who were there knew exactly how I felt and let me know they felt the same way, so that's the only way I knew I wasn't crazy. Having cancer is the same way. People who never had it just don't know what it's like. You need to talk to someone else who's been there, so you know they understand.[5]

Like Vietnam War veterans, many people with serious illnesses such as cancer believe that only those who have gone through a similar diagnosis and treatment can appreciate the experience of another patient. There are certain things that those who have not struggled with cancer will never understand; only fellow survivors can. Cancer patients need to find others who have had a similar experience. Cancer support groups can help fill this unique need to meet and talk with other survivors.

I hadn't been in a room with people who all had cancer before and I hadn't also been in a room with people my own age who had cancer. It was just very normalizing and such a relief, I can still feel it. I feel like I need to do that again! Lauren, age 22

Self-help groups are most helpful with problems such as feeling isolated or discriminated against, and with feelings of anger, self-blame, and guilt.[6] Members of self-help groups will sometimes say they feel they have no other place to get help dealing with these problems. We draw strength from each other when we realize we share a common bond. When we are able to listen and show understanding and compassion for one another, our groups become stronger.

The bottom line is that once a month I get together with a room full of women, all of whom have had breast cancer. And just the air in the room is a relief to breathe.[7]

The need for cancer survivors to regain control and to feel that we have the ability to make decisions about our lives might also help to explain why *self*-help groups – organized and led by cancer survivors rather than health-care professionals – are such an effective model for helping cancer patients. In self-help groups, cancer survivors themselves make the decisions for their groups. A self-help group is a truly "patient-centered" or "patient-driven" model of caring.

THE SELF-HELP MOVEMENT[8]

The rise of Alcoholics Anonymous and related self-help programs over the past fifty years and the subsequent expansion of mutual-aid groups to address a range of social justice and health problems can be seen as part of a larger effort by people with common and unmet needs to band together to help each other.

Since the 1980s the World Health Organization (who) has been supporting the development of self-help through workshops, publications, and recommendations. In December 1985, representatives from some thirty self-help clearinghouses throughout the United States and Canada met together for the first time in Texas. One result of the Texas meeting was the establishment of the International Network of Mutual Help Centers. The goal for the Network is to share information, resources, and ideas that promote awareness and recognition of the value of self-help groups.

The most important activities in the self-help movement take place at the local-community, grass-roots level. Most groups have very small and modest beginnings. Because of this it often takes a long time for a self-help group to surface. Self-help groups for cancer are no exception. The earliest report of a cancer support group was one founded by parents of children with leukemia in 1973.[9] The need has existed since long before 1970, but it has taken time for the movement to mature, especially because there has been little formal recognition of the value or benefit of this work, and little institutional support. The cancer support movement is part of a global trend to be more connected with our communities. People seek out others to help cope with fear and anxiety and to increase their sense of personal strength. Helping one another by drawing together through a crisis of cancer is an expression of a basic human need to belong with people in a welcome and safe community. We can expect that as long as cancer patients experience stigma, fear, and loneliness with the diagnosis, cancer support groups, and perhaps especially self-help groups, will continue to multiply, becoming permanent components of cancer care.

> *It gives me that space once a month for two hours where I'm looking at the whole thing straight, and I'm not playing games, and I can just relax. Whether I like these people or not is totally irrelevant. Because on the level of what I experience we share, I love them all. And we're all in the same boat.*[10]

The International Network of Mutual Help Centers has defined "self-help or mutual support" as "a process where people who share common experiences or problems can offer each other a unique perspective that is not available elsewhere."

They describe the characteristics of self-help groups as follows:

- Self-help groups are run by and for group members;
- Group activities focus on giving and getting support through storytelling, discussion, and sharing experiences;

- Self-help groups are open to anyone who shares the common concern;
- Self-help groups usually meet in person on a regular, ongoing basis;
- Groups are voluntary and open to new members;
- There is no cost except for small donations to cover expenses.

ARE THERE ANY RISKS OR LIMITATIONS TO SELF-HELP?

People who are not professionals sometimes worry about the *legal* risk of providing self-help. However, since self-help groups do not involve professionals acting in a professional capacity, legal risks are not an issue.

Nevertheless, there are several challenges that self-help groups need to be aware of. The most common challenges are "doctor-bashing," dealing with death and grief, stagnating or getting "stuck," focusing on negative attitudes, and depending too heavily on the group facilitator or leader. Problems such as these can happen when there is no facilitator or the facilitator has not yet developed skills or when groups lose focus, when the needs of the members change, or when there are members who dominate, bully, or try to take over the group.

Groups which have skilled group leaders or facilitators are best equipped to work through these types of difficulties. Facilitators need to have some general knowledge about cancer and the psychological issues faced by cancer patients and their families. Such facilitators are usually cancer survivors who also have some knowledge or experience with group behaviors and feel comfortable with people who have cancer at any stage of illness. This does not mean that group leaders must be professional facilitators, but they do need to have a demonstrated ability or training, plus a willingness to learn how to help self-help cancer groups work effectively.

Another concern is making sure that members are ready for a group. Some of us need to work through the adjustment to a cancer diagnosis on our own before being able to participate in a group. The spirit of self-help is that we come when we are ready, take what we need, and give according to our abilities.

Difficulties can also occur when new members join a group and are uncomfortable with frank talk about some issues, such as sexuality or fears about death. New members may expect unconditional optimism and decide not to return to the group if the meetings offer something else. Self-help groups can attract a variety of people, including some who have needs that a self-help group is not designed to meet.

One of the challenges for cancer groups and other self-help groups is to recognize the limits of what can be done. It is important to remember that self-help groups are not a good fit for everyone.

Groups need to know when to make referrals to other agencies and helping professionals. A support group is not a therapy group, and members cannot provide psychotherapy, medical care, or treatment. People who are suicidal or clinically depressed or suffering from serious mental illness need professional help. A self-help group *can* help direct people to find out about the appropriate resources. In this way, the group becomes part of a continuum of care that responds according to individual needs without trying to fill everyone's needs.

WHAT DO PEOPLE TALK ABOUT WHEN THEY GO TO CANCER GROUPS?[11]

The main reason people seek support groups is to get support. People want to learn how to live with cancer, and they believe that talking with people who are going or have gone through treatment will help. Most support groups provide at least some of what people hope for. Learning to live with cancer takes time and work. Groups help people who are newly diagnosed to understand that the ability to live with our illness comes to many of us with time.

Common themes that arise in support groups include:
+ learning to manage anger;
+ living with the fear of dying;
+ managing fatigue and pain;
+ coping with depression or guilt;
+ the search for hope;
+ the search for spiritual meaning in life.

> *I've often said that in one sense all the things we do – the support groups, the classes, the social events – are merely excuses to bring people together, structures in which that can happen.*

Discussions are not limited to this list, however. Members also discuss struggles with marriage or partnerships, sexuality, dependency, and loneliness. They talk about problems communicating with family, friends, and caregivers about treatments and prognosis. A lot of time is also given to concerns about treatment decisions, side-effects, pain, relationships with health-care providers, complementary therapies, and financial burdens.

Cancer support groups provide a place to talk about our own fears and to learn new ways of being. For example,[12] after the lengthy dying process of one member of a group, another member talked about her fear that her own death might be long and painful. Her oncologist and nurses and others who cared for her explained that no two patients are alike and that she should not assume that what happens to one of us happens to all of us. However, it was not until other group members brought up the fact that each of us has choices about our illness that she was able to see herself as different from the member who had died.

If you can talk to somebody who's been through it and have your questions answered honestly . . . what a relief. . . . we had one girl, she said, "This is better than winning the lottery. A meeting like this and getting all this information."

Whether the talk focuses on psychological issues or practical matters, participation in the group meets an underlying need for relief from fear and depression. Many people come into groups feeling isolated and lonely and somehow "different" from others, even loved ones. Expressing and sharing feelings helps people gain a sense of belonging – of being "normal" again. The sense of relief this provides is a critical part of the group's effectiveness. These are feelings that we often withhold from family and loved ones, because we feel a need to protect them from our fears about cancer. In the group, we find a safe, credible place to speak about these feelings, and to let them go.

I think the fact that other people have the same feelings . . . you're not a nut, that kind of thing. If you bite your nails for two weeks and are irritable and not fit to live with, and well, you learn that we all do it, so it seems.[13]

FOUR WAYS GROUPS WORK

In general, people in groups help one another in four ways:

1. by listening to others and telling their own story;
2. by sharing information based upon personal experience;
3. by offering emotional support through empathy and understanding;
4. by providing a sense of belonging to the group.

CHARACTERISTICS OF SUCCESSFUL CANCER SELF-HELP GROUPS

A group is effective when members understand one another's needs and can work together to try to meet them.[14] In successful self-help and support groups, members help each other rather than relying on a facilitator or leader. When a group is working well, members can sustain their feeling of connectedness to other group members even when they don't agree on issues. Ideally, a group culture develops and people feel a bond of intimacy, commitment, acceptance, understanding, and safety.

> *I think we helped each other more than the facilitator helped us, but I think her role was necessary because she kept us on track.*

Research[15] on the impact of self-help groups suggests that the more actively involved people are with their group, the more satisfied they are both with the group and with their own lives. These people report higher levels of life satisfaction, reduced use of health-care services and treatments, increased self-esteem, improved coping skills, and a more positive attitude towards their problems. Feelings of loneliness, fear, and confusion are significantly reduced.

IN THE TRENCHES: STORIES FROM CANCER GROUP MEMBERS

CONNECTICUT

I got a call from a nurse with the town health facilities and she said she felt there was a great need for some kind of support group for women with breast cancer because she was seeing these women all the time. Particularly the under-served or women that just didn't have any other kind of support system. She called me and considering the passion I have for these things, I said lets meet. And God works in funny ways because she is a terrific woman. She hasn't had breast cancer. She is a nurse that works with orthopedics but she has a lot of general medical practice experience. She is so committed to doing this that when we started together the passion just met and we started a group that to this day is very successful.

THE CANCER SUPPORT COMMUNITY, SAN FRANCISCO, CALIFORNIA (BY TREYA KILLAM WILBER):

CSC comes from a softer "we're in this together" kind of place. Yes, we believe techniques (visualization, meditation) can help, but we're much more interested in meeting people where they are and giving them what they ask for than in proving a point. In fact, I've often said that in one sense all the things we do – the support groups, the classes, the social events – are merely excuses to bring people together, structures in which that can happen. When I had cancer I found that it was difficult to be with my friends. I had to expend a lot of energy taking care of them, explaining things, dealing with their fears for me, with their often-unexpressed fear for themselves. I discovered that being with other people who had cancer felt like a big relief. I realized that I had become a member of another family, the family of people who know about cancer from personal experience. And I believe that much of what csc does is to provide a place and a way for members of that family to come together and support each other. Support each other through friendship, through sharing information, through sharing fears, through being able to discuss things like suicide and leaving your children and pain and fear of pain or death and what it is like to be bald and so on.

CHICAGO:

The telephone was ringing in Mimi Kaplan's living room and the news was not good. She had just returned from playing racquetball that day in May, 1977 and she recalled thinking to herself, "I feel great!." In fact, she wasn't great. Her doctor was calling and as soon as she heard his voice she knew. Breast cancer.

Once the shock of the mastectomy wore off and she learned two years of chemotherapy would follow, Ms. Kaplan was seized by terror. Not of cancer and not of losing a breast. How she wondered, was she going to cope with being a wife, mother, and university professor while undergoing chemotherapy. And, she had no one to ask. "Everyone kept saying, "You'll be fine. Just live as if nothing had happened,"." It didn't make sense.

Ann Marcou felt equally alone after both her breasts were removed in 1976. "Cancer patients have a life-threatening illness. Family and friends mean well, but they either avoid the issue or offer false assurances. I needed someone to talk to." A mutual friend suggested that Marcou, who was working on her master's degree in Therapeutic Communication at Governors State University, get in touch with Kaplan, who worked in the campus library and taught there. "I walked into the library, found Mimi and said, "Hi. I'm Ann Marcou and I've had a mastectomy." And we never stopped talking."

The two women discovered that beyond cancer, their biggest problem was finding people with whom to share their fears and answer the many questions resulting from breast cancer. What helps with nausea from chemo? Can I wear a bathing suit? Which prosthesis is best?

The answer to their questions, was Y-ME, a non-profit organization that Marcou and Kaplan founded in 1978 to offer counseling and fellowship to others. The program, their involvement and their feeling of accomplishment was the best medicine for Caplan and Marcou. "Y-ME has done more for us than it has done for the people we have helped,", said Kaplan. "When you have cancer, you're always living with the thought that you could die sooner than you expected. We wanted to leave something behind, something to be proud of." "And we are," Marcou said. Mimi Kaplan died in 1983 from breast cancer. Over 20 years after helping launch the organization, Ann Marcou continues to volunteer her time with Y-ME.

DO ALL SELF-HELP GROUPS WORK?

Not all cancer self-help groups are useful or effective for members, for a variety of reasons. Members may be too overwhelmed by strong emotions to be able to help each other. The group may be dominated by a member who is angry or bullying. The group may not have a clear focus or purpose, so that members don't really know what to expect. Or a change in facilitators or members may result in a loss of focus. Cancer self-help groups are run by and for people living with a life-threatening disease, and the people who volunteer are also struggling with illness and debilitating treatments. Stresses on members can result in group burnout from time to time. Such problems can be avoided if a group has skilled and competent facilitators, a clear purpose that is understood by everyone, and some simple agreements about how members will work together. Later chapters outline more detailed strategies for building and maintaining successful groups.

WHY SELF-HELP GROUPS ARE NOT PART OF STANDARD MEDICAL TREATMENT

The traditional medical approach to understanding illness and healing focuses on the individual patient not on what groups can provide to patients. Because health-care resources are limited, health services focus on treating the physical disease. Self-help focuses on meeting the emotional and spiritual needs of the whole person. Although there is still a perception that the effectiveness of self-help or support groups is unproven, there are now dozens of studies[16] in oncology that have shown improvements in patients' quality of life as a result of their participation in groups. There is an ever-increasing body of knowledge demonstrating the value and effectiveness of self-help. Eventually, this research, the demand for services by aging "baby boomers" affected by cancer, and the lack of funding for hospital-based supportive cancer-care services will combine to make self-help groups an increasingly routine part of treatment planning.

WHAT ARE THE DIFFERENCES BETWEEN SELF-HELP GROUPS AND THERAPEUTIC GROUPS?[17]

Self-help groups are different from psychotherapy groups in goals, leadership, philosophy, and a variety of other ways.

Goals: A traditional psychotherapy group focuses on personal change and understanding our resistance to change, rather than on support. The primary goal of therapy is to help people change something about themselves so that they can function better in relationships or other areas of life. Personal observation and reflection are expected from people in psychotherapy groups; supporting each other is not the primary goal. Support groups, on the other hand, help members find meaning and a sense of belonging through their participation in the group process. When this happens, people often change even though that is not the goal.

Leadership: Unlike professionally led therapy groups, self-help or mutual-aid groups have a facilitator who is not a professional leader. Self-help groups often get support from professionals, but the groups are led, or "facilitated," by a member or members who share the common problem of the other members. Support groups subscribe to the self-help philosophy that "helping others helps me." The facilitator's role is to promote group cohesion, provide information, remind members of the rules and structure they have agreed upon, and assist with appropriate actions when there are problems. Good facilitators help groups to function in a safe, welcoming manner.

Philosophy: The person asking for help is both an active participant and a helper in the process. By being the helper as well as the recipient of help, the group member acquires the enhanced self-esteem and feeling of worth that comes from being important to others.

Source of expertise: Professionals have credentials to show that they are trained practitioners of psychotherapy. In self-help, members' qualifications are their life experience, experience which is shared by all members.

Social distance: A professional must be objective, remaining detached from group members or individual patients; the self-help group member is both the person helped and the helper, within a close personal network in which members share strengths and difficulties.

Style: To receive formal services, a client makes an appointment, pays a fee, and continues therapy for a set, limited period. Self-help members are often available for practical assistance whenever the need arises, there are no fees, and the length of term is often indefinite.

HOW CAN SELF-HELPERS AND HELPING PROFESSIONALS WORK TOGETHER?

In the past, self-help groups have often been reluctant to work with members of the helping professions. More recently, however, as self-help has gained credibility, a number of self-help groups now want to have professionals involved, including as co-facilitators.[18] Research also shows that active involvement by professionals, either as consultants or to help a group get started, improves links among the various groups involved with cancer patients and strengthens the effectiveness of both self-help and professional approaches.[19] For example, having helping professionals involved with your group can make it easy for members to make appropriate referrals to meet a variety of needs. Members of cancer groups often have difficult emotional issues to deal with, and your group will want to know where to send people whose requirements exceed what the group can provide.

Group members who are in the helping professions, such as psychiatrists, psychologists, social workers, nurses, and therapists, need to make clear what they understand their role to be in the group. For example, they need to clarify whether they are contributing as professionals or from the shared experience of cancer.

As a simple guideline, the expression "on tap, not on top" may help to define the right partnership between self-helpers and professional helpers.

SUMMARY

- People who share common experiences or problems have special knowledge that comes from living with the problem.
- This shared knowledge creates a bond and makes group members uniquely qualified to help one another.
- Through active participation in the group, members can overcome their isolation and regain a sense of control.
- Leadership is shared.
- The goal of the group is to provide support for members learning to live with cancer.
- Shared experience creates a sense of safety in which hope for healing can grow.
- Professional partnerships are encouraged.

Thinking It Through Before You Start

To know what is happening, push less, open more and be aware.

The Tao of Leadership

2

The basic principles of the self-help movement are:

+ be brave;
+ start small;
+ use what you've got;
+ do something you enjoy;
+ don't overcommit.[20]

The underlying theme of the self-help movement is "self-knowledge." You need to develop a clear picture of your feelings, your goals, your skills and abilities, and the depth of your commitment before you embark on this undertaking. The exercises in this chapter are designed to help you do that.

STEP 1: THINK ABOUT YOUR OWN REACTIONS WHEN YOU WERE DIAGNOSED

Before starting down the path of self-help work, take some time to think about your own reactions to your diagnosis. You might find it helpful to work through the list of questions below with a close friend or family member.[21] The questions are designed to help you think about your own feelings, experiences, concerns, and needs, and about how your responses will help you when starting or facilitating a group. There are no "right" answers. This exercise is intended to help you clarify for yourself what and why you want to start up or help with a cancer group.

+ What did I think about people who had cancer before I was diagnosed?

- How did I feel when I first heard the diagnosis?
- Was it different from what I expected or wanted?
- What would I write in a note to someone facing a similar diagnosis?
- What is the worst part of the diagnosis?
- Who was the easiest person to talk to?
- Was I angry with the doctor? Why?
- What did I do about being angry?
- How has my doctor or nurse made me feel especially good or bad?
- How have people reacted?
- How did I deal with the loneliness?
- How did I deal with the fear?
- What problems have I overcome?
- What problems am I still struggling with?
- What were my dreams before the diagnosis?
- What are my dreams now?
- How has my life changed?
- I have learned something very special from my cancer experience. It is ...

STEP 2: CONSIDER WHY YOU WANT TO DO THIS WORK

You might also consider what you believe you have to offer other cancer patients and survivors – what your underlying aims are.

Which of these suggestions describes you?

- I want to share my experience with others.
- It helps me to know I am not alone.
- This work is interesting.

- My cancer has been treated and I am well. I feel obligated to give back.
- I am grateful for my health and want to tell others about the things that helped.
- I believe that support groups can help cancer patients to become well again.
- I want to be involved in something important.
- I want to return the kindness I had from others.
- Helping other people helps me.

STEP 3: IDENTIFY THE SKILLS AND ABILITIES YOU BRING TO THIS PROJECT

The personal skills inventory[22] is designed to help you set goals for your own development. You can answer the questions on your own, but it would be useful to do this with others who will be helping start the group.

Read through the list of skills and decide where you fit on the scale. Write down other skills you think are important. Then review your list and choose the skills you want to work on. Facilitating a cancer group requires skills in helping other people to express themselves, being objective and non-judgmental, helping the group stay focused, and respecting guidelines. Facilitators also need to be able to manage difficult behaviors without offending. If these skills are unfamiliar for you or if you realize that facilitating a group is not for you, there are many other ways you can help. You probably know someone who would be suited to this job. Ask that person about joining you or coaching you and other members in facilitation skills.

Personal Skills Inventory

Communication Skills	ok	need to do more	need to do less
Talking in groups			
Being brief and concise			
Drawing out others			
Listening generously			
Thinking before speaking			
Keeping my comments on the topic			
Not interrupting			

Observation Skills	ok	need to do more	need to do less
Being aware of tension in the group			
Being aware of the energy level			
Being aware of who is talking to whom			
Being aware of the interest level			
Sensing the feelings			
Being aware of who is not talking			
Being aware of anyone who is left out			
Being aware of the effect my comments have on others			
Being aware of issues the group is avoiding or being distracted by			
Being aware of silences			

Problem-Solving Skills	ok	need to do more	need to do less
Recognizing a problem			
Stating problems clearly			
Asking for ideas, opinions, and responses			
Giving ideas			
Summarizing the discussion			
Clarifying the issues			
Making a decision			
Implementing the decision			

Morale-building Skills	ok	need to do more	need to do less
Showing interest			
Getting others involved			
Creating linkages			
Getting agreement			
Ensuring a safe, democratic, open process			
Appreciating others' ideas and abilities			
Recognizing individual contributions			

Emotional Expressiveness	ok	need to do more	need to do less
Telling others how I feel			
Hiding my emotions			
Disagreeing openly			
Expressing warmth			
Expressing gratitude			
Being sarcastic			

Facing and Accepting Emotional Situations	ok	need to do more	need to do less
Facing conflict and anger			
Facing closeness and affection			
Accepting silence			
Facing disappointment			
Facing sadness			
Facing grief or loss			

Social Relationships	ok	need to do more	need to do less
Acting dominant			
Trusting others			
Being helpful			
Being protective			
Rescuing			
Needing attention on me			
Standing up for myself			

General	ok	need to do more	need to do less
Understanding why I do what I do (insight)			
Encouraging feedback from others about my behavior			
Accepting help willingly			
Giving feedback to others			
Criticizing myself			
Waiting patiently			

STEP 4: FIND OUT IF OTHER PEOPLE SHARE YOUR VISION

If you did this exercise with others who are interested in starting a group, you can discuss the results with them. If you have been working alone up to now and are eager to continue, this is the best time to start looking for people who share your interest and some of your values. You need to find others who are interested in starting (not just joining) a cancer self-help group. Working with others will keep you from burning out when the workload grows. But most importantly, when you have your first meeting and start sending out messages about what you are doing, it will be seen as a group effort and not just one person.

Finding other cancer survivors who want to do this work can be challenging, so here are a few tips:

♦ Tell the staff at the cancer-treatment center, clinic, or hospital about your idea and ask them if they know of anyone with a similar interest.

♦ Talk about your idea with family, friends, co-workers, and neighbors.

- Ask if you can post notices at the clinic, hospital, treatment center, or other places where cancer patients look for information.
- Talk to other self-help group leaders in your area.
- Find out if the local offices or chapters of established cancer organizations and charities have self-help services or training workshops. Ask how you can work together.

I love that Ken wants to have children. But who knows what my health will allow? But whatever happens, I suppose I will always consider things like the Cancer Support Community as my child. It's so special and like a doting parent I'm so proud of it.[23]

SUMMARY

1. Think about your own reactions when you were diagnosed.
2. Consider why you want to do this work (your goals).
3. Identify the skills and abilities you bring to this project (personal skills inventory).
4. Find out if other people share your vision.

Getting Started

The wise leader teaches more through being than through doing.

The Tao of Leadership

3

FIRST CHECK OUT THE TERRITORY

Although a few cancer support groups seem to get started and keep going without much planning, most need some help, especially in the beginning. It is a good idea for you and your co-planners to find out what is being done already. You might consider attending the meetings of an existing cancer self-help group nearby. Let them know what you are planning and ask for advice. Try to get a feel for how they operate – then borrow what you consider the best techniques and use them in your group.

A WORD OF CAUTION

Planning a cancer support group is not easy work. It takes time, and not all of the work is fun or interesting. As well, people will have different ideas about how much planning and arranging should be done, and how much administration or structure a group needs. For some people this will be stressful; for others it will be exciting. Taking the "we'll cross that bridge when we come to it" approach will usually help, but it can sometimes result in conflicts and disappointment. The planning, discussing, and conflict- or problem-solving stages are important for your group's development. Managing conflict and differences of opinion with respect and successfully negotiating agreements will be important parts of the learning process for your group.

UNDERSTANDING THE STAGES OF GROUP DEVELOPMENT[24]

Knowing something about the different stages of group development can help you cope with the difficulties that can arise. Whether your group is just starting or has been around for a while, the behaviors associated with the different stages may help you understand where your group is and what might happen next.

STAGE	BEHAVIOR
1. *Forming*	This is the beginning stage when people: ♦ get acquainted ♦ define their purpose ♦ lay ground rules ♦ begin to trust each other
2. *Storming*	This is the conflict stage when the group is sorting out differences, relationships, leadership, and power. The group begins deciding what to do next. If difficulties at this stage are not resolved, the group may disband. Disbanding is an appropriate choice for many groups when people can't reach agreements or when people don't have the time, energy, resources, or good health to carry on.
3. *Norming*	This is when a group really becomes cohesive. It is characterized by: ♦ mutual acceptance of group members and the role each has ♦ harmony within the group ♦ commitment to the group's goals and willingness to abide by its agreements

4. *Performing*	The group matures and is working well. Members have a clear idea of the purpose, and the group is helping members to get their needs met. The group has evolved effective and appropriate processes for:

  + solving problems
  + making decisions
  + resolving conflicts

5. *Adjourning*	The group decides to end. Members should be given the opportunity to:

  + express feelings about the loss of group
  + remember successes
  + identify problems
  + hear from other members about what the group meant to them
  + celebrate and say goodbye to others

A group will often move in and out of these stages; few groups just move straight through them. Again, there is no right or wrong way for groups to develop. Understanding and recognizing where your group is in this process may help you to realize that other groups have been stuck and have worked through it. Hang in there!

START KEEPING A GROUP JOURNAL

During the hectic start-up period, it helps if someone volunteers to keep a record of decisions and actions taken by the organizing group. Then, when your group is established, new members can understand what, when, how, and why decisions were made. Keep contact names and addresses of people who help. This is a good way to record the history of your group right from the beginning. You might even use this as a story if your group decides to publish a newsletter later on.

MATCH GROUP MEMBERS' SKILLS TO THE JOBS TO BE DONE

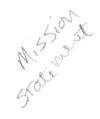

During the start-up or planning stage, your group will also be discovering the special skills that each member brings. If you have made a "Personal Skills Inventory" you probably have a good idea about each of your members' strengths, interests, and experience. A good rule of thumb in volunteer work is to match the person to the job. If someone in your group is confident and comfortable speaking in public, encourage her to be the spokesperson. Other members may have skills in writing, welcoming newcomers, maintaining computer data bases, phoning members, finding local resources, designing flyers, preparing refreshments, managing business details, or negotiating with professionals and businesses. When the job is satisfying, challenging, or rewarding, people will usually stick with it.

DEFINE THE PURPOSE OF THE GROUP

Determining goals will be one of the first decisions your group will make. A mission statement can help to define the purpose and goals. The mission or purpose shines as a guiding light, directing the members to stay focused on the goals and activities, and minimizing confusion and problems as the group grows.

For example, if a group decides its purpose is to offer education, new members will not expect socializing to be a major part of meetings. A cancer self-help group might have a mission statement such as *"To provide emotional support and information to people in our community who are affected by cancer.*" Defining the type of group lays the groundwork for all future decisions the group will make. A clear purpose will define the type of group, make clear to potential members what the group is about, and minimize misunderstandings about the focus of activities.

Once you decide the purpose, you will want to make certain it is clearly understood by everyone, including new members. Often groups will start every meeting by having a member of the group welcome everyone and explain what the group is for.

> Have clearly in mind what you want to say about the purpose of the group so that you are inviting the right people.

From time to time, when members are evaluating the effectiveness of the group, it may help to question if the purpose, needs, or expectations have changed. Again, there is no right or wrong way to do this. Members should be aware of changing needs and opportunities that come along and be prepared to respond to them.

ESTABLISH GOALS

Once the focus is clearly defined, group goals should be established. Goals emerge from the purpose and are usually stated as specific actions or activities of the group. One typical goal is to decrease the sense of isolation or loneliness people sometimes experience.

Groups can have many goals, including group goals and individual goals. If you don't know what cancer patients and survivors in your community need from a group, you might want to have a discussion about this as a part of the first meeting.

Individual goals might include:

- to deal with loneliness, fear, and isolation;
- to find a unique kind of support;
- to share experiences with others who are similarly affected;
- to share information about the services available;
- to provide a safe place to express feelings;
- to develop coping skills;
- to increase self-esteem.

Group goals might include:

- to learn from and provide encouragement to one another;
- to develop coping skills;
- to share problem-solving strategies;
- to overcome the stigma of a cancer diagnosis;
- to provide a focus when we feel confused and don't know where to begin;
- to explore non-traditional resources;
- to help members gain a sense of control;
- to provide relief for families and caregivers;
- to provide a safe, trusting, accepting place where confidentiality is ensured;
- to raise awareness about the needs of cancer survivors in the community.

Your group may find it helpful to discuss some of these goals and how they might apply to your cancer support group. Your list of goals may also help you describe your group to outsiders, or write about it in a newsletter, or advertise it in flyers or posters.

CHOOSE A NAME

Another important step will be choosing a name for your group. Naming your group and perhaps choosing an image or logo to represent your goals are another way of establishing your identity in your community. When naming a new group or revitalizing an existing group, facilitators need to involve members. The name and the logo can be used in newsletters or on flyers and other items such as T-shirts promoting the group. For example, a group of adolescents named their group Lasting Impressions. This name was chosen partly to make a humorous comment on the impact of chemotherapy, but more importantly to express participants' desire to be remembered and make a contribution, regardless of the length of their lives. The group also designed their own logo, two hands joined and enclosed in two circles, which is on a T-shirt given to each new patient joining the program. The logo visually communicates other group goals – such as emotional closeness and support.

Once the first steps are over, the members of the core group or organizing committee will need to determine if they want to continue their commitment and, if so, what role each person will play in the group.

GROUP MEMBERSHIP: THE BENEFITS AND CHALLENGES OF DIVERSITY

Some of the challenges and rewards of working in cancer groups come from learning about people's different life experiences, including:
   ◆ causes of illness and responses to treatment;
   ◆ beliefs about the role of health professionals and health practices in healing;

- attitudes about our bodies;
- past experience with illness or other health history;
- ideas about suffering, pain, and loss;
- beliefs about support systems, families, friends, professionals, and institutions;
- ways of caring and understanding who is responsible for caring;
- feelings about asking for support;
- ways of talking and expressing feelings;
- ways of working in groups;
- ideas about what is okay to talk about and what isn't.

If you want your cancer support group to be welcoming to all kinds of people, you will need to involve people from a variety of backgrounds and experiences. People at different stages of diagnosis and treatment will have different perspectives. Youth, seniors, men, and women will bring a range of experiences which will enrich your group culture. People with low income, men, gays and lesbians, elderly persons, and people from rural backgrounds do not use cancer self-help groups as much as others. Some research[25] found that about four times more women than men use cancer support groups. Other groups of people are also underrepresented in cancer support groups. People of color, low-income and elderly patients,[26] people with disabilities, and people in rural communities all face barriers to finding and attending support groups and professional therapy groups. Special attention should be given to making it easier for people in these groups to find the help they need and want.

Simple ideas such as serving food or organizing potluck meals are ways to get people interested in learning more about cancer groups. To attract people from minority groups, opportunities to discuss topics with a specific cultural relevance should be offered. One common theme for discussion in diverse groups could be ways of overcoming the stigma of both a cancer diagnosis and the need to ask for support.

People with young children may need help with childcare. With elderly cancer patients and survivors, providing transportation or meeting in a place that is close to buses and public transit, providing easy access for wheelchairs and walking aids, scheduling day-time meetings, and offering programs with a specific focus are important.

Ask members from different backgrounds and cultures what you can be doing to overcome any problems they might have faced in finding or joining the group. When you promote your group or when asked to do public speaking, be sure to invite members who represent diverse backgrounds to speak about their group experiences. If your group pays attention to being welcoming and aware of barriers, new-comers will recognize your genuine efforts to be supportive.

A word of caution. While it is important to try to meet the needs of as many people as possible, and while variety can greatly enrich a group, having members with diverse and competing needs can also add tension. Conflicts among members may arise when different groups of cancer survivors have different needs. There are no right answers or right ways to make decisions about needs. Members of support groups will need to consider what feels right for their group and be prepared for open and frank discussion.

In some cases, it may be appropriate to target a very specific group. People often find that the more they have in common with other group members the more comfortable and accepted they feel and the less time they need to spend explaining themselves. For example, young adults with cancer – aged 18 to 30 – prefer to meet with others of about the same age. They feel more able to share information about relationships, fertility, or sexuality among people who face similar challenges, though they may have different sites of cancer. Men with prostate cancer and women with breast cancer prefer to meet in groups specifically for their cancer types. Younger women often struggle to find a cancer group where they feel the other members share familiar concerns. People with advanced cancer or recurrence may also wish to be with people in similar circumstances. These groups are often part of larger groups, where all the members join together for the beginning and end of meetings, but break into smaller groups for discussion.

SUMMARY

1. Get started by first checking out the territory.
2. Learn about the stages of group development.
3. Start keeping a group journal.
4. Match group members' skills to the jobs to be done.
5. Define the purpose and goals for the group.
6. Choose a name.
7. Appreciate members' differences and make them work for your group.

Different Kinds of Groups and Group Structures

Learn to lead without being possessive.
The Tao of Leadership

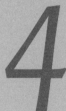

The feeling you want in a support group is informal, safe, and caring. And sometimes this spirit just happens. But most people involved with cancer support groups recommend working to achieve a balance between structure and flexibility based on your group members' needs and energy.

GROUP MEMBERSHIP

The needs of the members will determine the type of group. For example, women who have had breast cancer might feel more comfortable in a group only for women, while a group for newly diagnosed cancer patients who are having chemotherapy might welcome men, women, and young adults with any type of cancer.

One of the benefits of a group which includes people with all types of cancer, and perhaps also family members and friends, is that members see others in different stages of disease and learn how to cope with a range of problems. Generally speaking, though, it is harder to build cohesion and offer support when members share little except for a cancer diagnosis. The more people have in common, the faster they form bonds with each other and feel like part of a group. The common bond might be age, gender, cancer site, stage of illness, sexual orientation, or ethnic or cultural group. Having a lot in common increases members' sense of safety when talking about intimate issues such as sexuality.

> I think the fact that we were all young people was more of a commonality than anything else. I wouldn't have wanted to be in a group of people who all have the same thing. I wanted my cancer to be unique!

In some groups, the common bond may be that all the members are having chemotherapy, radiation, or bone-marrow transplant. Gender-specific groups are usually for women with breast cancer or men with prostate cancer.

MEMBERS AT DIFFERENT STAGES OF DISEASE

It is very important to think about whether meetings will be only for newly diagnosed people or will include long-time survivors or people with recurrence or progressive disease. Consider what might happen when newly diagnosed patients are in a group that includes people with metastatic or progressive disease. The newly diagnosed patient is typically hungry for information and needs encouragement about the opportunities for long-term survival.[27] On the one hand, being in a support group with a veteran patient who is struggling with advanced or terminal disease might be disruptive to building cohesion; but on the other, it may also give other members a sense of the seriousness of their situation.

Veteran cancer patients who have learned how to cope and who have made a positive adjustment to cancer – especially veteran patients who are living well with active disease – can inspire others to make difficult lifestyle choices. On the other hand, some veteran patients may not feel that the inexperienced, newly diagnosed patient can be much help to them. Or they may want to protect the other group members from sadness or fear of death.[28] Again, there are no right or wrong ways to decide who should be included in cancer groups. It is a question that each group must discuss and answer based upon the needs and abilities of the group.

Your group might begin to tackle this issue by starting with a simple statement. *"We are trying to create a group where people with cancer feel safe and welcome and are able to talk freely about living with disease. I am wondering how our group can be helpful to members who are at different stages in their disease. Do other members have any ideas about how our group can work for each of us?"*

The discussion will allow people to explore suggestions about creating a place for all members, even if that means some members may decide they want to meet separately for some of the time.

> *At one support group meeting, a woman talked about what it was like to live with a recurrence of her cancer. At the same meeting was a woman recently diagnosed, attending for the first time. After the first woman finished talking and group members had offered her their support, one of the facilitators said to the new member, "I imagine it must have been hard for you to hear this at your first meeting." This allowed a discussion about how both the listening and the telling can be difficult.*
>
> *One group was asked by a community hospice worker to consider if they could welcome a young woman living with advanced breast cancer. The facilitator's first thought was, "Oh no, don't send me anyone terminal!" She later realized she was overprotecting group members. The group had a discussion about it and decided to welcome the new member. One member said, "Would I not be welcome to come back to this group, if my disease progresses to the terminal stage? If someone wants to be here we should welcome her."*

If you and your planning group or members are struggling about what to do, consider asking a helping professional such as a social worker, nurse, or psychologist with specific experience in cancer patient groups to help you with this.

TYPES OF GROUPS

There are different kinds of cancer self-help groups, so planning will depend on what kind of group is needed in your community. Here are a few options to keep in mind.

TIME-LIMITED OR CLOSED GROUPS

Sometimes self-help groups will have time and/or membership restrictions, especially if they are affiliated with a hospital or treatment center. Each session usually has a prepared topic such as nutrition, treatment options, self-care techniques, and meditation. These are self-help groups if they are run by and for cancer survivors and the decisions are made by members. Such groups usually last from six to 12 weeks, and new members cannot start after the second meeting.

It can be hard to turn away people who come after the second meeting. However, members have an understanding that this is done to safeguard the sense of trust and cohesion that develops quickly. The focus is often on education or developing specific coping skills for newly diagnosed patients. Often these groups will have an experienced facilitator who is a veteran cancer patient; or the group may be co-facilitated by a helping professional and a cancer survivor. If the group is for a specific ethnic or cultural group, such as women of color or Native people, at least one of the facilitators or co-leaders must be from that culture. If a professional is asked to help the group get started, he or she will work in partnership with a member of the target group.

Closed groups can focus on learning a certain skill, such as those described in chapter 10, "The Healing Journey," or they can be aimed at providing support – frequently for newly diagnosed people. Closed groups often create a very safe and close-knit atmosphere for members very quickly. It may be easier to create safety and closeness when you know who will be at every meeting and how long you will be together. The members may also share a common interest in learning a new skill. Problems can occur, however, when the group ends and members have an ongoing need to stay connected.

At the end we just kept asking about funding – like, is there a way we could pay so that we could continue the group? All of us really wanted to continue the group after the time was up, but they said it wasn't possible. So we didn't. I have wanted to call them but it feels like a big distance now.

People who come to the closed or time-limited sessions may decide to come back again after the first group is completed or they may want to move on to an open-ended group that meets regularly.

OPEN GROUPS

These are the most common kinds of cancer self-help groups. Members meet on a regular basis – weekly, or once or twice a month – and follow a very informal meeting format. Although members may change from one meeting to the next, there is usually a core group who attend regularly. One or two of the group members will act as the facilitators, and other members will greet newcomers and returning members at the door. Other members may take care of phone calls, arranging the meeting room, newsletters, or publicity.

Often, guest speakers are planned, or decisions about business need to be taken care of, or issues need to be discussed with all the members. Meeting time is scheduled so that non-support issues are taken care of during a planned time period, but the group always keeps aside some time for talking together and sharing support. The purpose of the group is talked about at the beginning of the meeting, so that any newcomers will know what the meeting is about.

Open groups accept new members at any time, a fact that can be very helpful for people who are newly diagnosed and have urgent needs. As open groups mature, regular members often socialize more with each other, and the groups may become less welcoming for new people. Maintaining an effective open group requires occasional evaluation about how well the group is meeting members' needs. Groups that have a regular process for evaluation and that include frequent education or information sessions will be more likely to stay effective. The sample evaluation form on page 56 might be useful for your group members.

Although there isn't a lot of information that tells us if open-ended groups or closed groups are more effective in meeting members' needs, there is some evidence that cohesion, support, and mutual aid are more difficult to develop when members just drop in anytime. And, as mentioned earlier, research suggests that for men with cancer, the social support that is typical in self-help groups may not be effective for them. A more structured group which is time-limited and focused on education or providing information may attract more men members.

GROUP SIZE

Groups function most effectively for discussions when there are six to eight members. However, an acceptable range is from a minimum of five to a maximum of twelve members. When the group membership drops below four members, the group cannot work very well, and when it grows beyond ten members it becomes difficult to work on individual issues.

This doesn't mean your group shouldn't meet if there are not enough people – but you might consider finding another cancer group nearby to join with occasionally. That way your group will continue to have a separate identity but will have the benefit of learning from others from time to time.

EVALUATION OF SATISFACTION

Date:

1. How did you learn about the group?
   A friend / Referred by professional / Newspaper / Other

2. Is this your first meeting? Yes / No

3. Will you attend future meetings? Yes / No

4. Please rate the following aspects of the meeting:

	very satisfied	somewhat satisfied	not satisfied
Format of the meeting			
Length of the meeting			
Opportunity to talk			
Time of the meeting			
Location of the meeting			

5. How helpful was the group for you?
   Not helpful / Somewhat helpful / Very helpful / Extremely helpful

6. Describe briefly what was most helpful to you:

7. What did you get or learn from the group that you wanted to get or learn?

8. What did you like most about the group?

9. What did you like least about the group?

10. Do you feel any different about yourself after the group? Yes / No
    If yes, in what ways do you feel different?

11. Have you changed any behavior, ways or habits since participating
    in the group? Yes / No
    If yes, what has changed?

12. Please comment or provide suggestions for future groups and/or
    suggestions for improvement.

Reprinted with permission.
Guidelines on Support and Self-Help Groups,
American Cancer Society, Atlanta, Georgia (1994).

If your group meetings always attract more than twelve people, consider breaking up into smaller groups for the support discussion time. Your group will likely want to be all together for the opening and closing time.

KEY NEEDS OF GROUPS[29]

As we have said before, all groups are different and there is no one right or wrong way to go about starting or managing a group. However, to provide a genuinely "safe" place for members to bring their needs and concerns, every group needs to find ways to ensure the following:

- respect for differences;
- mutual trust;
- open communication;
- fair decision-making methods;
- shared goals;
- constructive methods of conflict resolution;
- maintenance of individual self-esteem;
- involvement of all members;
- attention to content (what is being talked about) and process (the way people are behaving, responding).

Some degree of structure can help to solidify the spirit of cooperation that makes the group a safe haven for all members. One member of a breast cancer support group that didn't have structure or a facilitator or guidelines about how the group would work reported,

Women were just complaining and crying, and one person was talking for a long time.[30]

AGREEMENTS

In fact, most cancer support groups find it helpful to develop a few simple ground rules that say how the group will function. Ground rules are created to provide a safe, informal, but structured environment for sharing and learning from each other. People attend support groups for a number of reasons, and simple ground rules will help ensure that each member's needs are addressed and that the group stays focused. Agreements define acceptable group behaviors and may be used to prevent offensive comments or actions, and limit constant complaining.

Agreements or norms can be drafted by the facilitators when the group is getting started and then shared with all group members. At the first meeting the facilitator might say,

> *To get the most from our group, we need some ground rules or agreements to help us relate to each other. Some that other groups have used are: starting and ending on time; speaking one at a time; sharing thoughts but not having to talk; and keeping things that are said in the group inside the group.*

With agreements, the facilitator does not have to be punishing or authoritarian but instead reminds members of the agreements acceptable to the group as a whole. If the group is open-ended, the facilitator should review the agreements at every meeting for the benefit of new members. The facilitator can ask a member to review the items agreed upon.

New members might have suggestions for adding to the list if other members feel comfortable with the suggestions. Try to keep the rules simple and easy to remember so that you don't need to write them down. Your group is trying to create intimacy and a welcome place. Don't go overboard with rules or you will turn people off.

I try not to push people to move in directions I have chosen or think I might choose myself.[31]

If your group does not have any agreements and you are having difficulty staying focused or are experiencing problems with difficult members, it might help to have an open discussion about developing agreements. Some suggested norms or agreements include:

1. The content of support meetings is confidential. What is discussed in group stays in group. No identifying information is to be shared outside of the group.

2. Group members do not judge one another. The purpose is both to give and to get support and information.

3. Members give their attention to the person speaking. One person speaks and everyone else listens. There are no interruptions or side conversations.

4. Members will speak from personal experience and not relate the experience of others.

5. Members will not pressure or oblige others to discuss feelings or experiences.

6. Meetings will be held on a regular basis, in a non-smoking, accessible, and convenient meeting place. There are no fees.

7. The group begins on time and ends on time.

8. Members are free to come and go without obligation to attend meetings. However, members are encouraged to give feedback to the group when they choose to leave.

CONFIDENTIALITY AND ANONYMITY

In an anonymous meeting, people are given the option of not revealing their names. In some instances, this may become very important if members are concerned about safeguarding information concerning their diagnosis. Other groups will not be as concerned about this, but there has been stigma associated with cancer for many years, particularly in some cultures.

HOT TIP

The exception to the rule about confidentiality is that confidentiality cannot be maintained when there is a threat of self-destructive or suicidal behavior. Should something like this happen during a group meeting, members can talk privately to the person and make appropriate referrals, as well as notifying family or friends, preferably with the knowledge of the person making the threat.

Confidentiality is the practice of keeping private what occurs and is discussed during a meeting. Since members often interpret this idea in different ways, it is important to define what your group wishes to keep confidential. Most groups ask members to say nothing outside the group about what was seen and heard in the meeting. Some groups practise a less strict degree of confidentiality. They allow members to talk about the meeting with people outside the group as long as no identifying information is used. Still other groups have no need for confidentiality.

This rule applies to the support group meeting, but of course if you invite the public to participate in an educational evening or fundraiser, you want people to talk about what they have heard.

FORMAT

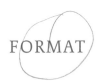

Creating a group environment that reinforces a climate of warmth and closeness suggests that the members maintain a consistent meeting time, place, room, and seating arrangement. A circle of chairs without any obstructions works best for everyone to see one another. More importantly, members will feel involved and part of the whole group. The facilitators should also attempt to have a similar format for beginning and ending the meeting. For example, many groups use check-in to begin meetings – the facilitator talks briefly about his or her own cancer experience, then invites members to give their diagnosis, an update about themselves since the last meeting, and a brief statement about what they hope to get from the meeting. If this is used to start each meeting, new members will become comfortable with the format and feel less anxious about future meetings.

"check-in"

Some cancer groups intentionally set a slow pace when starting up and before developing any structure. Talk with other members and the planning committee about allocating appropriate amounts of time for business, education, support, open discussion, program planning, and so on. Having a specific focus or topics which provide ongoing learning opportunities for members will help prevent your group from becoming stagnant.

STRUCTURED FORMAT

Structured groups usually have a set agenda with a prepared topic, followed by questions and discussion with all members participating. Members choose the topics and arrange speakers.

Research[32] tells us that men prefer cancer groups with a structured program and an emphasis on information and education. Formal presentations related to cancer diagnosis, treatment, and side-effects will usually work well and keep members interested. If the group focuses exclusively on information and education, however, it may be too easy for members to avoid expressing their feelings. Meetings need to provide some balance between time for information and time to discuss the emotional, spiritual, and social impact of cancer.

> *The matter of support had become an important item on our agenda. So the men decided that there would be a second meeting and that is where we feel the understanding and the warmth and we are free to talk when we want to.*

UNSTRUCTURED FORMAT

These kinds of groups usually have a brief "check-in" where members take turns *briefly* introducing themselves and stating what they hope to get from the meeting. The group will often have co-facilitators who help keep members involved and discussions on track. Usually the discussions are spontaneous, and any issue can come up. The facilitators need some group skills and guidelines to prevent the group from being overwhelmed by emotions or inappropriate behaviors.

SUMMARY

1. Think about group membership, including how to manage newly diagnosed people and people at other stages of cancer within the same group.
2. Decide what type of group (closed or open) is most suitable for your members.
3. Make some simple guidelines or agreements for working together.
4. Decide on the format (structured or unstructured).

Organizing Your First Meetings

The leaders presence is felt, but often the group runs itself.

The Tao of Leadership

5

Many cancer groups begin with a meeting that is open to any member of the public before having support meetings. This first public meeting should include *some* brief support time, because helping has to start right away or you will lose people. When writing flyers or promoting the meeting be sure to state that the meeting is to talk *about* starting a new group and that you will be planning the first meeting for group members to take place at a later time.

PUBLICIZING YOUR GROUP

Cancer support groups are not always easy to launch, and reaching potential members may take time. Some ideas for publicizing your meetings include:

♦ Put announcements in the (free) community-calendar sections of the local newspaper

♦ Send notices to radio or cable-TV stations.

♦ For underserved populations, put notices in the newsletters, cultural centres, grocery stores, schools, and churches that serve the people you want to reach.

♦ Meet with the staff at clinics or medical centers and talk with them about your ideas.

♦ Talk to community leaders who represent other cultures.

Don't be surprised if people are slow to respond to your invitation. It will take time and effort to build new relationships.

Whether your meeting is to launch a new group or you are providing information about your regularly scheduled cancer support group, try to keep the message simple, friendly, and welcoming. The message should include:

- ◆ WHAT the purpose of the meeting is.
- ◆ WHO is invited. Is it for cancer patients only, or also for family members, friends, and the general public? Is the meeting for people who are newly diagnosed or for anyone diagnosed at any time? Is it for a certain kind of cancer, such as breast cancer or prostate cancer? Does this mean women only or men only? Can doctors, nurses, or other care providers attend?
- ◆ WHERE the meeting is being held. Give specific and clear directions to the meeting room. A large, simple map is a good idea.
- ◆ WHEN the meeting is. Give the starting time and the ending time – and then make sure you start and end on time. If you plan a social time following the event, put this in the poster. That way, people who are arranging for someone to pick them up won't miss out on anything that is planned.
- ◆ Provide the contact person's name (first name only) and phone number.

FIRST PUBLIC MEETING

If you are starting with a public meeting to discuss the idea of a new group, your purpose will be to generate interest in your idea and find people who want to join or who want to help the group get going. Be sure and invite staff from cancer treatment centers, clinics, and surgeons' offices – they are often the ones who will refer cancer patients to your group. This kind of community meeting can serve several purposes:
- ◆ It brings together the people who want to work on cancer issues.
- ◆ It helps you to find out about other related services.

- It provides information to the general public about the support needs of people with cancer in your community.
- It helps you learn what people with cancer want in your community.
- It generates interest, energy, and enthusiasm.

There are, of course, many details to consider when planning a first meeting – such as finding the right location, getting the word out, creating print materials or gathering educational materials, booking a speaker, and so on. Each member of your organizing group might take on one or two of these tasks.

TARGET YOUR MEMBERSHIP

If your group plans to be closed and time limited such as an eight- to 10-week skills and education group, you need to tell people who can attend, when the membership becomes closed, and why. Give some thought to who can join and why.

If your meetings are for cancer patients and survivors only, think about making arrangements for family members or friends to meet in a separate place, away from survivors. Plan for when these people can join together and share some of the meeting time at the opening or closing. Caregivers have important needs, but survivors often have difficulty being open with friends and family in the same meeting. Separate meeting areas for these different groups will allow both caregivers and survivors to talk openly.

One prostate cancer group plans meetings that begin with members and partners or wives all together and then divides apart for some of the meeting. This allows discussion to flow freely without concerns that one partner is guarding or burdening the other.

Be aware that in some cultures women do not attend meetings without their husbands or partners. If you are targeting women from

66

these cultures, arrange the meeting to allow the family member, husband, or partner to be included.

FIND A SUITABLE MEETING PLACE AND TIME

Try to get a free space – the local library, church, community center, or social service agency. Try to avoid the hospital or treatment center if possible. Most cancer patients and survivors prefer to go to these places only when necessary. Try to find a place that is wheelchair accessible, accessible by public transit, and has cheap or free safe parking.

Consider the people you want to reach when deciding the time and place. One organization sponsors lunch-time support groups in the downtown business district to serve working women. If elderly cancer patients are the people you want to reach, consider day-time meetings along convenient bus routes that are well lit and within safe areas. Meetings should not last more than one and a half to two hours. It is also easier for people to remember the meeting time if it is held in the same place and at the same time each month, like the first Monday.

FINDING A ROOM

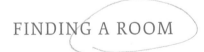

Most meeting rooms are not perfect, but a meeting space should be:
* comfortable (If a room is too hot or cold, or the chairs are hard or too low, or if there is noise or people wandering through the space, it will be very difficult for people to pay attention, much less share feelings or intimate stories!);

- clean, safe, non-smoking, and well lit at night;
- private;
- large enough to move around in without bumping into one another, but not TOO big;
- available long term;
- with access to convenient, clean washrooms.

Before deciding on the room, check on:

- keys: Who is responsible for locking up?
- room set-up: Do you have to arrange the chairs and other things before or after the meeting?
- availability: What hours can you have the room? Does everyone have to be out at a certain time? What about meetings that go on longer than usual or members who linger and chat?

Whatever space you decide on, it might be useful to have at least the first few meetings at the same place in order to build familiarity.

WHAT TO BRING TO MEETINGS

Supplies you may need at meetings include:
- a pad of paper or sign-in sheets with space for names, addresses, and phone numbers;
- pens;
- direction signs to use inside the building, if needed;
- name tags, reuseable if possible (use first names only);
- a flip chart, paper, and markers;
- flyers or brochures;
- refreshments – if your members agree.

AT THE FIRST MEETING

At the first meeting you will want to ask people to leave their names and addresses if they want to be part of the cancer support group. If the next meeting for the support group has already been planned, hand out flyers with date, time, and place.

TIPS

Here are some tips to consider before both the first public meeting and the first support group meeting:

- If possible, attend similar meetings beforehand, or talk with cancer survivors and patients who have organized similar meetings.
- Be there early to welcome participants. Your organizing committee should be ready to answer questions, give out name tags, and introduce people.
- Have a table set up near the entrance with some refreshments and print materials, brochures, newsletters, or articles you want to share. Ask people to sign in if they want to be contacted by the group after the meeting.
- Arrange the chairs in a circle if possible, so that everyone can see one another. Eye contact encourages communication. Leave an opening in the circle for people to join in easily.
- Start on time. It demonstrates respect for people who show up on time.
- Keep the spirit informal, warm, and welcoming. This is not a business meeting or a professional meeting. The first impression is important and should reflect warmth and caring for people.

- Keep the purposes of the meeting in mind: to connect with others who are living with cancer; to encourage everyone's ideas about what the group should be and do; and to set the stage for shared participation, respect, and open communication.
- Put together a meeting plan or agenda and write it down on a flip chart ahead of time. Post the agenda where everyone can see it and ask if anyone wants to add to it. Then be ready to change the agenda if the audience wants to add ideas. Remember, the agenda is just a guideline. Don't rush along just to cover all the items. The goal is to generate discussion, not to win the agenda race.

A SAMPLE AGENDA FOR THE FIRST PUBLIC MEETING

- Welcome the audience and introduce yourself and others.
- Explain the purpose.
- Invite discussion, questions, and answers.
- Summarize discussions and clarify agreements that are made.
- Let people know what will happen next.
- Say thanks and close on time.

We often have quite an extended coffee break of 30 to 40 minutes during which some very valuable conversation happens.

SAMPLE FORMAT
FOR A SUPPORT GROUP MEETING

Self-help has to start from the first meeting or you will lose people. When people first come to a cancer self-help group, they are often feeling very vulnerable and hopeful that the group can relieve some of the fear and uncertainty they have been dealing with on their own. Often, the need for support and information is overwhelming for people if they haven't been able to find someone to talk with. The cancer support group meeting may be the first time that the person has talked openly about diagnosis and treatments. The core group or organizing committee will have to be ready with a plan for the meeting.

Meeting Plan

1. Start the group on time and get going.
2. The facilitators should introduce themselves and let the group know what the role of the facilitator is. Remember to keep your story brief and on topic. This provides a model for other members on how to begin.
3. State the goals and purpose as defined by the core group or from the public meeting.
4. Let people know what the structure will be, whether it will be open-ended with members coming and going or a closed group with a time limit and new members starting and finishing together.
5. Have the facilitators explain the group's norms and agreements .
6. Invite members to contribute to the group discussion. For the first meeting, you might suggest a specific topic, such as coping with the diagnosis, and ask members to respond.

7. Think about a name for your group. A name will give your group a public identity. As well, the process of choosing a name together will help members to get to know one another and develop decision-making skills.

8. Do not try to deal with organizational issues such as leadership, fundraising, incorporation, and so on at the first meeting. Keep the focus on support.

9. Close by recognizing the value of the meeting. A brief go-around or check-out, with each member using one word to describe his or her experience, or just standing together in silence for a moment can be simple and effective closing rituals.

10. Serve refreshments before or after if your group agrees, and allow members some time for informal socializing before leaving.

Note: Not all groups want to have refreshments. It can be distracting if people are moving around or eating during discussions. Also, it can create problems if there are allergies or cultural concerns about food. Juice, tea, coffee, or water might be enough. Members can decide what suits your group.

FREQUENCY OF MEETINGS

How often your members meet will depend on their needs and the availability of facilitators. Weekly meetings reinforce cohesion and continuity, especially for newly diagnosed patients or those undergoing weekly treatments. For people who have a recurrence of cancer, frequent meetings may help meet a strong need to be with others who are facing a similar situation.

In rural areas, too, where the group may be the only source of support, frequent meetings may be helpful. For some groups, once a month is sufficient, but for others, meeting once a month may make members feel disconnected and needing to spend time getting reacquainted every month. Meeting twice a month is a compromise that can help members stay connected and allow new people to join in quickly.

CHILDCARE

It may be difficult for people with small children to attend meetings. If your group has funds, and members need help with childcare, you might try to arrange to provide care in another room during the meeting.

Make sure people call ahead of the meeting time so you can plan for the number of children needing care. Make sure the people caring for the children are capable and known to the group, and that they know where the meeting is being held.

TRANSPORTATION TO MEETINGS

Advertising your meetings well in advance is very helpful to people who have to arrange buses or rides or childcare. Members may be able to help one another with driving. The facilitator can raise the question during the business portion of the meeting or at the end of the meeting. Let members know the easiest route to your meeting by public transit.

EXPECT UPS AND DOWNS

Starting a group can be a very rewarding job that inspires lots of enthusiasm in the people working on the project. But it may also be discouraging when there are problems you hadn't planned for. And there are always surprises!

Your group will go through changes in attendance and energy. It's natural with all groups and you should expect it. Especially when members are struggling during treatments, attendance will depend on individual energy as well as group energy. Don't be discouraged. Support groups require a lot of work to start and maintain. Find other self-help group facilitators and ask if you can help each other by calling and meeting socially once in a while to offer advice and encouragement.

Ending your meetings on a positive note with an invitation for each member to comment on something good that they have gotten from meetings can help remind the facilitators of the valuable work they are doing for the community.

SUMMARY

1. Target the people you want to come to the meetings.
2. Find a convenient time and place.
3. Develop a meeting plan.
4. Develop an agenda.
5. Expect challenges.

How to Keep
Your Group
Working Well

Pay attention to silence.

The Tao of Leadership

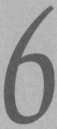

FACILITATION: THE SELF-HELP LEADERSHIP STYLE

The facilitators of a cancer support group have the challenging task of striking the right balance between encouraging candid discussion among all members who want to talk and maintaining a safe, welcoming environment. Facilitators usually have several roles, including:

+ promoting cooperation and cohesion;
+ developing a safe climate;
+ helping support evolve;
+ encouraging and showing appreciation for supportive efforts by members;
+ fostering stress reduction;
+ providing information;
+ encouraging discussion;
+ keeping members on topic;
+ reminding members of agreements;
+ helping with periodic evaluation and planning.

In short, facilitators illuminate what is happening by linking members' experiences, coaching members in problem-solving skills, and encouraging and inviting reflection and recognition.

CREATING A SAFE, EFFECTIVE GROUP

To develop a *safe* group climate, facilitators:

+ help members to accept and appreciate each other's differences;

- respect members' right to limit self-disclosure;
- use humor to balance and moderate intensity.

To maintain an *effective* group, facilitators help support to happen through education and by encouraging members to work together to reinforce positive and productive behaviors. They help relieve stress by planning for laughter and fun to balance the seriousness and by providing a structure that gives the group direction and support. A positive focus – learning about changes in diagnosis, treatment, research, and prevention; developing coping skills; inviting guest speakers with expertise – encourages growth. Without growth, a group may stagnate and become stuck. One sign of stagnation is that, while members keep coming back, they socialize and share friendships rather than being focused on cancer. If this happens in your group, it is time to re-examine or evaluate the group's purpose.

Facilitators should be well informed, but they shouldn't feel they need to have all the answers. Ideas are best explored with all group members. Facilitators help others to feel welcome and comfortable. They might seldom talk during the group meeting, but their presence helps all of the other members to do the work of the group.

CRITERIA FOR CHOOSING A FACILITATOR

Evaluations[33] from successful cancer support groups have described some of the characteristics of effective facilitators.
These characteristics include being:
- accepting
- active

- aware
- caring
- confident
- fair
- involved
- sensitive
- understanding

Many very good groups are led by people who have a natural talent for making a group feel warm and welcoming. They have common sense and good hearts and courage. Those are the people that you will find in your group by listening and looking at how they behave and how others react to them. The criteria for selecting the facilitators might also include searching for someone who:

- understands the difference between a self-help or support group and group therapy;
- is prepared to promote an atmosphere of acceptance and understanding;
- is able to promote the development of trusting relationships between group members;
- is a good listener;
- demonstrates a positive attitude towards his or her own adjustment to cancer and is able to be objective;
- has training or demonstrated ability to facilitate groups;
- is willing to continue learning, accept feedback, and promote evaluation.

Effective cancer support groups often have co-facilitators and shared leadership responsibilities.

DIFFERENT KINDS OF GROUP FACILITATION

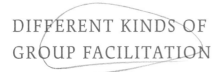

ROTATING FACILITATION

One way to ensure that the leadership is shared in a cancer group is to rotate the job of facilitator. This allows all of the members to share in the responsibility of managing the work of the group and to gain different perspectives on what the job requires. Your group can plan who will lead the meeting on which date for several months in advance. Be prepared to be flexible, however. Group members' health and other commitments may change and you will need to have a back-up plan in place. Using co-facilitators (see below) as well as rotating facilitation would mean that another person would be prepared to take over if one facilitator is not available.

SHARED OR CO-FACILITATION

With shared facilitation or co-facilitation, two or more people take on the facilitation tasks and roles. This type of arrangement is very popular with groups that decide to keep the same facilitators for a long period of time. There are many benefits of using shared facilitation:

- Each facilitator brings different strengths and skills to the role.
- Two facilitators can more easily ensure that both content and process are being attended to.
- Co-facilitators can learn from each other.
- Co-facilitators can provide encouragement and support for each other.
- Having a co-facilitator to share tasks and confer with after meetings helps prevent burnout.

Co-facilitators often plan meetings beforehand and discuss how the group went afterwards. Talking after group gives the facilitators a chance to discuss what was said and done, how they might handle things differently, and what can be planned for the next meeting. It is also a time for each facilitator to get and give support and encouragement, as a way to prevent burnout and fatigue.

Leaderless Groups, or All Members Facilitate

This type of facilitation usually works best for groups that have been together for some time, so the members know each other well and have developed a high degree of trust and comfort. In this kind of group, members have agreed about what they want to do at each meeting and they just do it. New members are welcomed and the process is explained. Most importantly, there is little conflict and high agreement about *how* the group works. Each member models appropriate behavior for new members, and all members practise facilitation skills. This type of facilitation is rewarding for groups who are committed to equal sharing and where there are shared values and styles. Many people like this informal and intimate approach as long as they are able to welcome new members into the tightly knit atmosphere.

In this model, the members all share in the tasks of the group by:

+ using questions such as "Has anyone else in the group had to deal with this?" "Would someone like to talk about how their relationship was affected?" in order to encourage open communication and participation;
+ respecting silence;
+ trying to stay focused;
+ trying to be flexible when surprises occur;
+ modeling compassion and supportive behavior by being non-judgmental, respectful, and accepting of feelings;

• helping with problem solving rather than focusing exclusively on negative feelings.

Some of us will be more comfortable with sitting back and listening and watching the way in which each member is reacting and contributing. Others may have identified personal skills that will help with the subject being discussed. Members need to draw upon their experiences in groups to know where their particular skills are and to apply them as either facilitator or group member. The Personal Skills Inventory from Chapter 2 lists some of the skills members can use to facilitate self-help groups.

A GROUP JOURNAL

No matter which kind of facilitation your group decides to use, it is helpful to keep a journal or a brief record of meetings. The information that is recorded should not identify members and should respect confidentiality and any other norms and agreements of the group. This record is an important history of your group's activities and decisions and will be very helpful to new facilitators.

HOT TIP

You should talk about the role of the facilitators at the beginning of each meeting for the sake of any new people. This will help everyone to understand that the members all share responsibility for the success of the meeting.

Record decisions made, norms and agreements, special guests or speakers, and any significant discussions. Quotes can also be important, but again, respect confidentiality. Let the group members know that a brief record is kept and that they are welcome to read the notes at any time.

TASKS OF THE FACILITATOR

In a self-help group, all members are regarded as equal and each member contributes. The group as a whole will need to make sure that the meetings stay focused and work on the goals. The leader of a self-help group does not direct the group in the usual ways of a group leader. Instead, he or she senses the group's direction and helps to guide discussion towards a constructive resolution. The facilitator is tuned into members and helps each person achieve goals. The facilitator is not controlling or directing but is attentive to the needs of the group, especially the need for a safe, compassionate environment.

Some specific facilitators' tasks are:
   ♦ to make sure meetings start and end on time;
   ♦ to help set the agenda;
   ♦ to help keep the discussion on topic, according to the agenda;
   ♦ to help set guidelines or agreements and to remind members of them, if necessary;
   ♦ to suggest a periodic review or evaluation;
   ♦ to keep a journal or record about meetings;
   ♦ to model compassion and supportive behavior;
   ♦ to share information;
   ♦ to take part as a member of the group.

Developing good group skills takes a lot of time and practice. Don't be discouraged if there are problems. Mistakes happen. People with cancer share very strong emotions, and group meetings can be rocky. Staying open to learning from mistakes helps the group maintain safety and trust. Practise forgiveness and good humor with yourself and other members of the group.

Ask other facilitators, cancer group leaders, or helping professionals for their ideas or suggestions, and problem solve together. Share what you learn with the other members of your group. They too want the group to work well.

CONTENT AND PROCESS

It is important for facilitators to keep track of what the group is discussing (content) and the way the members are interacting with each other (process). Having two group members act as co-facilitators can help to ensure that both the content and the process are being attended to.

By identifying for members what is happening within the group, facilitators can help bring the group back to a positive focus when members become overwhelmed with negative emotions or one member seems to be taking over the meeting. This does not mean that a cancer support group should never talk about negative or sad issues. Cancer support groups cannot take away the pain or suffering of a cancer diagnosis. However, it is important to find a way to bring the members through a difficult discussion in order to be able to end on a constructive note, since the purpose of the group is to help members to learn to cope and adjust to life after a diagnosis of cancer.

Group processes that facilitators might identify and use to help
bring meetings to a satisfactory conclusion include:

+ discovering shared feelings or experiences;
+ releasing tension through expressing feelings;
+ giving and receiving support and help;
+ sharing information;
+ working toward new insights;
+ learning how others cope;
+ bonding as a group;
+ developing a common sense of purpose and/or meaning.

Ways in which facilitators can use their awareness of process to meet
challenges that arise in the group are discussed further in Chapter 7.

FACILITATION SKILLS:

*Over the years, I've talked to a lot of people who have cancer, including
many who have recently been diagnosed. At first I wasn't sure what to
say. It was easiest to talk about my own experiences as a cancer patient,
but I soon saw that often that was not what a particular person needed
to hear. The only way I could discover how to help someone was by
listening. Only when I heard what they were trying to say could I
get a sense of what they needed, of the issues they were confronting
at the time, of the kind of help that would really help at that
specific moment.[34]*

Becoming an empathetic listener is a learned skill that is taught by
many volunteer or social service organizations. This is a skill that

cancer group members will find they need to use frequently, and one that is useful in all of our relationships. Consider investing time in getting this training, and encourage anyone who wants to take on the role of group facilitator to become trained. Ask your local non-profit organizations and social service agencies who train volunteers if they offer programs in active listening, or look in the "Resources" section of this manual.

> *The most valuable thing we can give another person, is the quality of our attention.*
>
> Dr. Richard Moss

ACTIVE LISTENING DEFINED [35]

To be an effective listener requires us to be present with the speaker with all of our body, mind, heart, and spirit. When you can hear the words and become aware of the speaker's body language, gestures, tone of voice, facial expressions, and changes in emotion, you are actively listening. In this way, you are able to follow along with the speaker, without needing to offer advice or comment. You are attentive to all of what you are hearing, not what you are thinking. Seldom in life do we have the experience of being heard in such a focused manner. The effect on the speaker of having your complete attention can often be profound. To be heard, to be accepted without judgment, is a wonderful gift to give and to receive.

> *I believe I listen well, and I have a good deal of trust in people, a lot of confidence that people bring with them the resources to cope with life as it touches them. Which means I don't need to solve things for them. I can listen, and I can then ask if there is someone in the group that is able to relate to this person, and so that is the real work of the group.*

Active listening is a way of communicating that helps clarify another person's way of thinking. Most of us are in the habit of listening to others, but active listening is more than just hearing words. Active listening involves using skills that enable the listener to understand meaning. It means paying attention to the speaker's use of specific words, the meaning of the words used, and the feelings and actions that go along with the words.

People diagnosed with cancer often feel very threatened and defensive. They may feel that they have lost control of their life. Often they develop a negative self-image. Active listening allows people to talk and explore their self-image knowing that the listener fully accepts them as they are without reservation or expectation. Active listening promotes personal growth and helps strengthen a person's sense of self. The good listener provides:

- non-critical acceptance;
- a genuine sense of equality and freedom to speak;
- understanding and warmth.

LISTENING FOR MEANING

Since people go through so many different phases during the course of an illness that can be persistent and unpredictable as cancer, learning to listen to what they need is especially important.[36]

The content of the message is a statement that tells you what the problem is. The feeling or attitude underlying the content often conveys the speaker's true meaning. For example, when a speaker says, "I just found out I have cancer and I'm very upset and confused," *having cancer* is the content and *upset* conveys the feeling of the message. Often, the content is not as important as the feeling underlying the message. Start with paying attention to the feelings, and encourage the speaker with open-ended questions. By listening you will be able to help the speaker recognize his or her feelings. Only when the speaker is fully aware of those feelings and able to manage them will he or she be able to understand any explanations or information.

Many people remember very clearly the moment they heard their cancer diagnosis, but few of us remember anything else after hearing, "It's cancer." Everything else is just noise.

Noticing Cues

Much of our communication is non-verbal, so it is important to pay attention to the other messages we get from such things as body language, hesitation in speaking, tone of voice, mumbling, avoiding eye contact, shifting about in the chair, and so on. All these help convey the total message.

Clarifying or Paraphrasing

Because understanding what a person is really saying can be quite difficult, it is important to test your understanding. You can do this by restating in your own words what you believe the speaker has said. Check out with the speaker if your understanding matches the intended message. An example of such checking out might be to say, "If I understand what you are saying, Jim, you haven't been talking to your family because you want to protect them. Now you are angry because they aren't being very supportive. Did I understand that correctly?" Wait for the other person to clarify if your understanding is correct. Don't be surprised if there are long silences while the person reflects on what to say next. Try not to interrupt the silence or hurry the person to get an answer; silence can be more effective than speaking. Remember, your goal as the listener is to check out the intent of the speaker, not to give advice or make judgments.

Empathizing

Empathizing is not simply saying, "I know how you feel." It is trying to understand another cancer survivor's experience in the way he has described it. To empathize is to "tune in" to another person's emotions and feelings expressed through words, body language, and movements. Allow the speaker time to fully express herself. Allow the speaker to become aware of feelings and to begin dealing with them. Be present with your body, mind, and heart and try to resist the temptation to be distracted with your own solutions and thoughts.

Empathizing Versus Sympathizing

Being sympathetic means feeling sorry for someone. When we offer sympathy, we are not on an equal footing with the person we are listening to or helping. Our feelings of pity will be obvious. This response will not likely be helpful and, in the long term, the person may regret having shared intimate and vulnerable emotions with you. Empathizing keeps the listener on an equal footing with the speaker, recognizing the uniqueness and dignity of the speaker's experience.

Using Silence

Many of us are not comfortable with silence and feel the need to fill the void. Silence can be a very effective tool when used with skill and awareness. Silence can help slow down discussion and allow group members to gather their thoughts. It can have a calming effect on members who may have become frightened or whose thoughts are scattered.

> If there is silence, let it grow. Something will emerge. Let the storm rage; there will be calm.
>
> Tao Te Ching

While a prolonged silence can create negative feelings or make members wonder if there is a problem, it is important not to be too anxious to re-start discussion. Timing is important. Generally the listener should respect the silence and allow the person to resume the conversation when he or she is ready.

ASKING OPEN-ENDED QUESTIONS

Open-ended questions, such as "Can you talk about how you would like the group to help with this problem?" require the person speaking to expand on an idea or comment. Open-ended questions invite the person talking to continue the discussion and explore difficult or complex issues knowing that the listener is willing and interested.

A closed-ended question, such as "Can we talk about this at the break?", can be answered with a simple yes or no and may be helpful if you need to stop someone from talking. Try to limit the use of open-ended questions when you are coming to the end of the meeting time.

VALIDATING EXPERIENCES AND STRENGTHS

When someone tells you his or her story, you can show that you have listened by affirming the messages the person has conveyed. For example, you might say, "It sounds as if that conversation with your daughter was really important for you," or "It took courage to say what was in your heart." Even when stories are hard to talk about, you can affirm the strengths that people have shown.

BRIDGING OR LINKING

Facilitators and other group members can use bridging or linking to help new people to connect with the group and each other. The opportunity to make such connections is one of the most important benefits of belonging to a group. Your group will develop a more cohesive and intimate group spirit through the highlighting of common experiences. It can be comforting to learn that other cancer survivors have had to face similar problems and some of the same feelings, and that they have found ways to cope. This technique requires some skill, a good memory, and careful attention to confidentiality. For instance, when a member talks about problems with understanding treatment choices, you might remember that this came up at a previous meeting. You can say, "This is something I recall talking about earlier. Does anyone else recall that discussion?"

RESPONSES THAT STOP PEOPLE FROM TALKING

Try to discourage *"Why?"* questions. Such questions can sound judgmental or blaming. For example, the question "Why did you go to *that* doctor?" makes it sound as if the patient is responsible for getting poor treatment.

> *A dear friend of mine, who made me feel beautiful even when my hair fell out, recently said, "You didn't choose what I would have chosen, but that didn't matter." I appreciated her for not letting that come between us at what was clearly the most difficult time of my life.*[37]

Other responses that inhibit speakers rather than help them include:

- changing the subject;
- not making eye contact;
- being easily distracted – answering the phone, reading, turning away;
- questioning decisions or making judgments;
- giving advice or offering opinions;
- constantly asking the speaker to repeat what he or she is saying;
- interrupting;

- showing pity;
- rescuing;
- being glib or philosophical;
- rushing the speaker.

To summarize,[38] active listening involves behaviors and attitudes. An easy way to remember them is the formula BRIEF:

B *body posture*, including movements and gestures which communicate awareness;

R *respect* for the other person's right to speak and be heard;

I *intimacy*, which requires a safe, caring environment in which ideas and feelings can be freely expressed without fear of judgment;

E *eye contact*, which communicates interest and attention;

F *following*, which is both verbal and non-verbal. Verbal following includes the use of open-ended questions and minimal words. Non-verbal following includes nodding, smiling, and appropriate facial expressions.

MAKING GROUP DECISIONS

Important decisions are seldom made by one person in self-help groups. This is because self-help groups place a high value on the involvement of members in all matters that affect the group. Keeping the administrative needs of your group simple will limit the kinds of decision-making problems that you face.

MAJORITY RULES

This is the most common method of group decision-making. Issues are discussed and, if more than half the members agree on one thing, the decision is made. This can be useful when there is little time for making a decision and with issues where consensus (everyone agrees) is not possible, although a dissatisfied minority will remain. It can be effective when the decision made is not a critical one.

CONSENSUS

Most self-help groups strive to attain consensus when making decisions that are important to the whole group. Such decisions include what the purpose of the group is, who the members are, and when and where to meet. Everyone should have an opportunity to influence the final decision. The consensus model can work only in groups where the members basically like and trust one another, however. Otherwise, differences of opinion will not be valued, but will be seen as threatening. The advantage of a decision made by consensus is that practically all members will be committed to it.

Many groups aim for "modified consensus." In this model, the group may be close to full agreement and those who disagree may go along with the rest of the group when they know that their opinions have been heard. It can take a lot of time and energy to achieve consensus – everyone needs to be heard. As well, consensus rarely occurs, since there will often be as many points of view as there are members. But for the important decisions, attempting to reach consensus is very useful. The process brings group members together and ensures greater commitment to carry through on the decision.

SUMMARY

1. Choose a facilitator and decide on the style of facilitation.
2. Keep a journal of meetings.
3. Understand the job of the facilitator.
4. Practise active listening.
5. Understand how to make decisions as a group.

Challenges
Facing Groups

When a person is calm complex events appear simple.
The Tao of Leadership

In cancer self-help groups, as in most groups, there will be challenges. Members can learn how to become effective at confronting problem behaviors or difficult members without offending, and thereby become less dependent on the facilitator to handle issues. Members will also improve their own sense of self-esteem and competence when they learn how to manage problem situations.

MAINTAINING MEMBERS' SELF-ESTEEM

Understanding how cancer affects self-esteem may improve the ability of group members to help one another. When our self-esteem is threatened by illness, our behavior can become difficult for other people to cope with. We don't necessarily want to be threatening or frightening to others – especially people who might be able to help – but illness can cause us to be very defensive and not act our best.

Self-esteem is a measure of how we feel about who we are and how much we enjoy being who we are. People with high self-esteem don't always feel good about what is happening to them – such as a diagnosis of cancer – and they might want to change their circumstances. But they don't want to become someone else. Positive or high self-esteem is a good foundation for mental and emotional health. People who go through life with low self-esteem may often feel as if something is wrong or missing in their lives. Because we live with ourselves all the time, it is important that we enjoy our own company, or we will always be looking for something or someone else to make us happy.

A person's sense of self-esteem can change frequently. When our life changes for the better or the worse, our level of self-esteem moves up and down. High self-esteem is like a bucket full of water; we can dip in and draw from the bucket without noticing that we have lost anything. But if we have lived with low self-esteem for a long time, another drop out of the bucket can leave us feeling completely empty. The effects of cancer and its treatments can have a powerful effect on our sense of self-esteem.

There are many sources of self-esteem. We will discuss four. The first is recognition, or being valued and cared about, particularly by those who know and love us. When we go without it, our self-esteem is lowered just a bit. Recognition can be a warm hello or hug from a family member. It can also come from having the boss ask how we feel. But when we have cancer and are in treatment, the change in daily routine means we often don't see the people who give us recognition. Or we see them so much, they forget to acknowledge us.

A second source of self-esteem is a sense of achievement, accomplishment, or mastery. Long-term accomplishments often have to do with major goals such as marriage, raising kids, building a business, being promoted, going to school, staying in good physical shape. Short-term achievements may include such things as keeping the house clean, mowing the lawn, preparing a meal, or participating in sports or family activities. Cancer and cancer treatments can leave us feeling sick or exhausted and unable to do these things. Again, not being able to feel the sense of accomplishment we usually get from such activities will affect self-esteem.

A third source of self-esteem is having a sense of control, influence, or power over our lives and the way we lead them. Having a sense of power comes from being able to make choices and arrange for things to happen the way we want them to happen. Having cancer and needing to take treatments will mean having to make clinic appointments and spend time in hospitals or treatment centers. Cancer can interfere with travel plans, weddings, planning a family, school, careers. We lose the ability to control how we spend our time – at least temporarily. Of all the four sources of self-esteem, having a sense of power and influence seems to carry the greatest weight; it can take us down and build us up faster than the other sources.

A fourth important source of self-esteem is our personal values and beliefs. These values and beliefs are unique to each of us. What we value is often based on a belief or a combination of beliefs. Personal values and beliefs can be based on spiritual or religious experiences, or can be bound up with family, work, education, relationships, sports or fitness activities, art, or music. Our ability to act on our personal values helps us to maintain our self-esteem. If religious belief is important to us, being able to attend services or prayers will help us maintain our self-esteem – especially after a diagnosis of cancer. Being unable to play music, practise sports, or participate in a regular exercise program will have a negative impact on self-esteem for people who value these activities.

If members are missing the recognition they are used to receiving from significant people in their lives or are not feeling cared about, the group can encourage them to recognize and ask for what they need – for a phone call, perhaps, or to be touched or hugged. To enhance the sense of achievement or accomplishment, members can encourage one another to take on small tasks. Even small accomplishments will increase self-esteem and stop the downward spiral of negative thinking.

Encouraging people to find out about treatment options is an excellent way to help them regain a sense of power and control. Working with them to prepare a list of questions or helping them find their way through the confusion of the cancer clinic can boost people's self-confidence immeasurably.

Encouraging people to explore alternative ways of living by their personal values and beliefs can help people find their way back to doing the things they value. When they are ready, managing personal hygiene, preparing a meal, walking or other moderate exercise, going to church, or listening to music are simple ways to increase self-esteem.

One last comment on self-esteem. For some of us, being a cancer patient can become a source of power and increase our self-esteem as a result of what are referred to as the "secondary gains of illness," such as the special recognition, support, and sympathy of family and friends, or the time off from work and other duties. But although we might be tempted to use our cancer experience to exploit the good-will of others, we shouldn't confuse having cancer with being worthy of love and attention. Being worthy of the love and attention of others has to do with being and acting in loving ways and appreciating others. The best course is to nurture good relationships – both when we are sick and when we are well.

STRATEGIES FOR COPING WITH DIFFICULT BEHAVIOR

"It was hard to have a conversation with anyone – there were too many people talking."

Yogi Berra

At some time, every group will have someone whose behavior causes problems for other members. A list follows of some of the most common problem behaviors and suggestions for how to cope with them.[39]

THE MONOPOLIZER
This person needs to tell his or her story at every meeting and in every discussion, and wants all of the group's time and attention.

What to try: First, acknowledge this person's needs. Then try to redirect his or her energy. A person who is new to the group or newly diagnosed may be very needy of your group's attention, but you shouldn't allow the behavior to continue at every meeting. Explain the guidelines and agreements that help members to be respectful and share time. If this does not work, for the sake of other members it may eventually become necessary to ask the person directly not to monopolize the meeting. Give the person the choice of continuing with the group and respecting agreements and the needs of other members. If the person is unwilling to comply, privately ask him or her to leave the group.

The Help-rejecting Complainer
This person complains all the time but refuses any helpful suggestions, using expressions like "Yes, but" a lot.

What to try: Group members can confront the complainer and build on the positive experiences that everyone in the group shares. Focus on things that can be done. Ask specifically what the complainer was hoping to get from the group. Remind the person that the group can only be effective when members actively participate and are genuinely committed to learning. A self-help group is not a captive audience for people who need to complain endlessly, without making any effort to accept responsibility for the things they can change.

The Hostile Member
Unlike people who use anger to mobilize themselves into constructive action, the hostile member directs anger at other members of the group. This kind of person may also be very hostile outside the group as well.

What to try: Actively protect the safety of the group by setting firm limits – respect for other members, no interruptions, no judgments. Make sure the hostile member understands the agreements and norms. If the person will not or cannot conform to the group rules, privately ask him or her to leave. Again, the safety of the group is more important than an individual's need to rage.

THE WITHDRAWN MEMBER
This person rarely or never talks or participates in the group.

What to try: Encourage participation. Watch body language carefully and try calling on the person when you notice signs of a response – for example, if the person's eyes light up during a certain discussion, or if the person nods when someone else is talking. Use check-in times at the beginning or end of the meeting when everyone says a few words to help him or her connect with the rest of the group. Support and encourage everyone's participation but don't demand it. Good listeners are as valuable to a group as those members who regularly speak.

MEMBERS WITH MENTAL HEALTH PROBLEMS
People who are suicidal, psychotic, or deeply depressed do not usually do well in cancer support groups, unless their mental health condition is under control.

What to do: If the condition is obviously a problem, refer the person to mental health services or groups. Let the person know that when he or she is ready, group participation may be appropriate. Remember, there is a clear difference between self-help and mental health services or therapy. Some people will need help that is beyond your group's ability, and you need to refer them to the appropriate professionals.

The problem behaviors described here can threaten the spirit and effectiveness of the group. When the facilitator and other members confront the problem behavior and set limits, group members can feel confident that problems will be resolved. This allows the group to grow and continue to be effective, safe, and welcoming, recognizing that the welfare of the majority of members must be protected.

ASSERTIVE CARING

Assertive caring is an approach to managing problem behaviors that is very effective for self-help groups. Anyone can learn this approach and, with some practice, this will help facilitators and members to prevent difficult members from taking over a meeting.

In *The Self-Help Leader's Handbook: Leading Effective Meetings*,[40] the authors describe assertive caring as a way to say no without offending. It involves providing a statement of understanding, setting limits, suggesting an alternative, and checking for agreement.

Assertive caring can be used with a range of types of difficult behavior, including:

- ◆ when one member of the group talks too much;
- ◆ when one member interrupts frequently with irrelevant and/ or inappropriate remarks;
- ◆ when a member responds with "Yes, but" to everything suggested by other group members;
- ◆ when a member consistently arrives late and/or interrupts group meetings;

- when a member appears to need more help than the group can give;
- when a member has significant problems that other members do not share;
- when a member makes discriminatory or offensive remarks.

THE THREE STEPS IN ASSERTIVE CARING

1. *Provide a statement of understanding:* For example, if a group member is taking up a great deal of time with the same problems at each meeting, you might say, "I understand you are having trouble getting help from your husband and family since your diagnosis."

2. *Set limits:* Let the person know why you need to change the situation. You might say, "Many of us have struggled with our families' reactions. I know I did. We have spent time in our last meetings exploring many options with you. But right now, we need to let other people have a chance to talk."

3. *Suggest an alternative and check for agreement:* In checking for agreement you need to make sure that the suggestion is acceptable to all the members. You might say, "Perhaps you could continue talking about this after the meeting. Would that work for you?"

Of course, assertive caring won't work in every challenging situation. If the situation is more complicated, the whole group may want to brainstorm alternatives. It is important to be flexible and caring, and to find solutions that don't embarrass or show disrespect for the group member.

WHEN A FACILITATOR IS DOING TOO MUCH

When all eyes are focused on the facilitators much of the time, or when the facilitators are doing most of the talking and answering all the questions, they are doing too much. Again, the role of the facilitator is *to make easy* the work of the group, *not to do* the work of the group. Members have to be involved and responsible for what happens in the meetings or the group will not work. If members always look to the facilitators to answer questions and solve problems, they will not have the experience of solving problems for themselves. The following steps may help the facilitators avoid becoming overinvolved:

1. Keep the opening remarks welcoming, brief, and on topic.
2. Do not respond right away, even when questioned directly. Make sure others have a chance to respond first. If support is needed, members may wait for a moment before offering it.
3. When no members are responding to questions, try to draw members in by using open-ended questions such as "Has anyone had any experience with this problem?"
4. Schedule regular evaluations to ask about the role and skills of the facilitators and invite suggestions about needed changes.

PREVENTING FACILITATOR BURNOUT

Sometimes I feel that I've gotten in over my head. I don't begrudge it, but sometimes I'd like a whole week where I don't have to think about cancer.

Burnout is a serious problem with no easy solutions. However, you can work to organize your group so that no one is unduly stressed. A few suggestions for preventing burnout follow:

1. *Suggestions for the group as a whole:*
   - Develop structured guidelines. Some groups develop specific guidelines on how to handle difficult situations or problem behavior. This policy can relieve the facilitators of some of the worry about how to handle difficult situations.
   - Have more than one or two facilitators and rotate the job every few meetings.
   - Limit the length of time people are expected to serve. Imagining that your job as facilitator will never end can cause burnout.
   - Practise saying thank you to the facilitators at every meeting! Celebrate and reward facilitators at least once a year!

2. *Suggestions for facilitators:*
   - Write down your feelings and comments in the diary or notebook you keep for the group. De-brief with your co-facilitator after meetings as a way of giving and getting feedback and support for your efforts.
   - Find a helping professional in your community who will support you in a "coaching" or mentoring relationship. Professionals can provide valuable help with problem solving, referrals, and other support.
   - Bring in new group members and prepare them to do facilitation. Register them for appropriate training or skills workshops. Coach the new facilitator, then ease your way out.
   - Let your group know when you start to feel overburdened. You too are a member, and sharing your feelings with other members is what it's all about.

Do's and Don'ts for Facilitators[41]

Do	Don't
Participate	Take over
Provide information	Lecture
Encourage everyone to talk	Pressure
Empathize	Focus on yourself
Clarify people's feelings	Prevent members from doing so
Let members explore feelings	Rescue people
Protect members from hostility	Block expressions of anger
Support and balance different views	Take sides
Prepare an agenda	Insist on following the agenda
Use structure and predictability to reduce anxiety	Substitute structure for control
Acknowledge group tension	Avoid tough issues
Use humor to reduce stress or bring people together	Use humor to distract or avoid
Encourage members to explore questions	Assume you need to have answers

SUMMARY

1. Understand how self-esteem affects behavior.

2. Recognize common challenges in groups.

3. Practise assertive caring.

4. Take steps to prevent facilitator burnout.

Grief, Loss, and Bereavement

A knowing leader takes time to nourish self as well as others.

The Tao of Leadership

8

Being a member of a cancer support group requires courage in facing fears about our own death and dying. We come together in our groups and find other "veteran" cancer survivors who share their experience, strength, and hope. We breathe a sigh of relief because at last we have discovered someone who has walked in our shoes. We start to regain our own strength and sense of control from the veteran cancer survivors – believing that if they can do it, so can we.

But there will be people in the group whose disease gets worse – not better. And there will be deaths among group members. The effects of these losses and deaths on group members can be devastating, especially when members have also become friends.

This presents a dilemma for the cancer support group members.[43] On the one hand is the desire to maintain a hopeful attitude and not overwhelm new members with stories of loss and grief. On the other is the desire to extend support to members who are dying and to grieve for the friends who have died. In cancer self-help groups that are unable to meet the needs of seriously ill people there is often anger, both from the person who is ill and from other members who wanted to be more helpful.

> I was going to bring up the issue of S's death and how we had not dealt with it, and I really felt badly because I didn't go to the funeral because I was too much of a coward. But the gal who was newly diagnosed was sitting three people from me, and I just couldn't bring it up. I didn't know enough about her, and who would be at home for her.[44]

By now you may be thinking that starting or joining a cancer support group is not such a good idea. Maybe you are thinking it will be too painful or remind you too much of your own fear of death. This is especially true if, like most cancer survivors, you are still struggling with your own grief at various losses – the loss of your sense of immortality, your health, your sexuality, and so on. Perhaps, like most cancer survivors, you would prefer to maintain a positive attitude and stay away from people who are really ill, maybe even dying. After all, most survivors want to put cancer behind them and go on with their lives. Again, only you can decide what is right for you.

If you choose to join a cancer support group or start a new one, you will have an opportunity to be with people through some of the most difficult and rewarding days of their lives. But you don't have to face this difficult subject alone. There are many helping professionals who can guide you in learning how to become comfortable with people at all stages of disease.

Learning to be with dying people in a way that enriches life can help groups to grow and become more authentic. This is not to say that groups become expert at this. But when members find the courage to be with one another and talk openly about death, they also find comfort and relief just from being together in this way.

This chapter is about understanding how a cancer support group can help not only members whose cancer is getting worse and whose life is ending, but also those who are worried about how to discuss fears about death and dying and those who are grieving the losses they have felt because of their cancer diagnosis.

Your greatest teachers will be the members of your group who struggle with this most difficult challenge. Your group cannot, of course, take away anyone's pain or anger or sadness. But they can offer a safe place to express those feelings by being accepting of each person, at whatever stage of illness.

> *When I talk to someone who's been newly diagnosed with cancer or who has a recurrence or who is growing tired after years of dealing with cancer, I remind myself that I don't have to give concrete ideas or advice to be of help. Listening is helping. Listening is giving.*[45]

You and your group members will also discover courage and compassion within yourselves that will help you on your own journey. Although there are some skills you can learn to help prepare you for this work, experience will become your best teacher. The more you are able to face these difficult issues with a willing mind and open heart, the more able you will feel talking about death and loss.

If your group is just getting started or if you are currently struggling to support a dying member and your group is feeling overwhelmed, help is probably available right now in your community. Churches and funeral homes often have staff who are trained in bereavement counseling. Hospices and groups for bereaved families have people they can call on who are experienced in dealing with death and dying, and they may help you find someone who can meet with your group. The right person can become an ongoing resource to discuss with your members how to be helpful to others, how to cope with projections about their own death, and how to use rituals and ceremonies to remember and celebrate the life lost.

There is no easy way to do this, and there is no right or wrong way. But having an understanding of the process of grief and healing can be helpful for facilitators and other group members.

MANAGING GRIEF AND TRANSITIONS

Grief is a highly personal and normal response to a life-changing event. It is also a process that can lead to healing and personal growth. Groups can help provide support during, after, or in anticipation of loss. Such help can include companionship, understanding, practical help, a safe place to share feelings, or a place to talk away from overburdened family and friends. The group can offer a safe place to draw feelings to the surface, so we can move towards healing, no matter what the outcome of the disease.

FROM LOSS TO HEALING[46]

Any loss that causes a significant change to our lives is a life loss. Death is the most obvious life loss, whether it be the death of group members, parents, children, relatives, friends, or colleagues. But other losses can also be wrenching and cause pain or grief. These can include the loss of a relationship, job, pet, home, or business; or of health, mobility, or memory. The loss of a breast or limb or the loss of bowel or bladder control from cancer will be a life loss. The loss of our sense of youth and immortality is common after a cancer diagnosis.

The future we had hoped for, our self-esteem, our sense of control, of meaning in life, of identity, of belonging, even our sexuality are often changed or lost to us. In other words, on the inside we might feel as if we are going crazy. One of the most common expressions we hear from bereaved people is, *"I thought I was going crazy."*

When we grieve or mourn these losses, we experience feelings of powerlessness, fear, anger, and guilt. At the same time, we are aware that society has many taboos about expressing such feelings. Certain unwritten but definite and potentially harmful rules take effect. These rules or myths can come from friends, family, the workplace, even the cultural or religious community. Some of the rules are:

1. Don't talk about it.
2. Don't feel, cry, or show emotions; you will upset others.
3. Don't trust. This one comes from inside the person who is grieving when that person accepts the first two rules. ("If I cannot feel or talk about it, whom can I trust with my feelings, my story, my urge to talk about my loss without fear of rejection or judgment?")

4. Don't think for yourself. ("They know best. Who am I to question them?") Grief can make us feel helpless and unwilling to trust our own knowledge and instincts. We believe that others know more about what is good and right for us than we do ourselves.

5. Don't change. This is the most dangerous of all. Change is threatening to those around us, because if we can change, then they will have to change. But if we don't change, we won't grow or heal.

So there is pressure from inside – we can feel crazy. And there is pressure from outside – the rules. What can groups do to help? Cancer support groups help break old rules and create new ones. In cancer support groups we can:

- find a safe place to talk and to tell our story;
- help our fellow members to recognize and manage today's reality;
- learn to think for ourselves and regain some sense of control;
- celebrate changes and milestones and life, no matter what the outcome.

Change is certain. Growth is optional.

TRANSITION CYCLES

The following chart illustrates the flow of emotions and different stages that people move through in the grief process. It is designed to help you understand what some of the common responses are during the different stages and how group members can be helpful. Not everyone experiences all of the stages, and people do not necessarily move through them in precisely this order. Rather, we may move randomly between stages as a result of different influences.

DENIAL

Reactions:
  numbness
  feeling overloaded
  anger

Group responses:
  comfort
  support
  encourage expression

COMMITMENT

Reactions:
  re-create future
  start decision-making
  seek symbols of
    remembrance
  take risks

Group responses:
  support
  recognize
  celebrate

TRANSITION CYCLES

RESISTANCE

Reactions:
  low energy
  confusion
  loneliness
  pain

Group responses:
  identify sources of
    support
  remain calm

EXPLORATION

Reactions:
  begin to recognize
    that death does not
    destroy love
  become able to listen
  begin to regain power

Group responses:
  comfort
  validate
  explore options

RITUALS AND CEREMONIES

Mourning is a process we go through to help us undo our connection with whatever we have lost. Mourning helps us to move forward in our grief. The rituals that are associated with mourning, such as funerals, burials, and wakes, have roots in the cultures and communities we come from. When we experience illness, aging, or a life crisis, these life events awaken a need for meaning in our lives and we often reach back to our family, culture, or community to help us.

Rituals help us to recognize, validate, and honor the meaning in each life. Our ancestors recognized the intimate relationships we humans have with nature. They recognized rhythms in the natural world around them. They honored the flow of life and death and marked the cycles of change. In doing so, they believed they helped one another to grow and change. Rituals can help us to gain a sense of being connected to others and reduce our sense of confusion and isolation. Meaningful rituals offer a sense of comfort, peace, and acceptance in difficult times.

Group rituals may be as simple as lighting a candle at the beginning of the meeting, standing quietly in a circle, or taking turns speaking from a book of poetry or affirmations. Checking in with each member at the beginning and end of the meeting is also a form of ritual. A ritual is any practice or behavior that is repeated in the same way at the same time and that has special significance for those who perform it. A ceremony is usually more formal and not performed as frequently. One cancer group holds a yearly ceremony to celebrate the lives of members who have died and to honor all of the members who volunteer time for the group. Families and friends are invited, candles are lit, and members read aloud the names of all of the members who are being remembered and honored.

Some groups incorporate special props or activities into their rituals or ceremonies, such as:

+ quiet music, drumming, bells, gongs;
+ songs or chants sung together;
+ candles (not in a laryngeal cancer group);
+ poems or special readings;
+ stones, feathers, shells, or special objects that are passed to each member.

When a person is born, we celebrate; when they marry we jubilate; but when they die we act as if nothing has happened.

Margaret Mead

Many groups have found that rituals are a way to help members recover from loss and grief as well as to celebrate success. To develop and practise rituals requires courage, vision, humor, and creativity.

Meaningful rituals and ceremonies touch us in all parts of our being – physically, emotionally, mentally, and spiritually, and they can help to nurture our healing and sense of well-being. Avoiding or not talking about death or loss can be as painful or difficult as struggling through the discussion. Talk with other groups about how they remember members who are dying or who have died. Consider talking with a bereavement counselor or social worker or nurse with experience in helping people who are grieving.

GUIDED IMAGERY

Some groups use visualization, or guided imagery, as part of their ritual or routine. If this is a new practice for your group or if new members are not familiar with using imagery, you could start by explaining that the exercise is used to "help shift gears, get focused, let go of the business of the day, and get comfortable being together." For guided imagery to be effective, participants must be relaxed.

If you are planning to use this with your group, you will probably want to practise first at home with friends or family or with a tape recorder. During the exercise, speak much more slowly and with longer pauses than you usually do. Remember that your listeners are forgiving – if you miss the words or get tangled up, slow down and repeat the words. It helps to begin in a similar way each time. An example of a guided imagery session follows. You may wish to modify it to suit your own style.

GUIDED IMAGERY

Start by helping group members to do some simple relaxation exercises, focusing on relaxed breathing. Then proceed by saying:

"Make yourself comfortable on your chair. Take off your shoes and place your feet flat on the floor, about shoulder width apart, hands open and facing upwards, resting on your legs or knees.

"Gently close your eyes. Begin to pay attention to your breathing. Notice the rhythm beginning to slow. As you breathe in, feel the energy begin to fill your body with a quiet vitality. As you breathe gently out, notice the release of stored tension. Feel your face, mouth, and eyes relax, your shoulders and neck drop and become heavy. Notice that your breathing is soft and quiet.

"Now imagine yourself in a place that is familiar. It is a place of comfort and safety and beauty; it is your own sanctuary. You have visited this familiar and warm place before; you are welcomed again by the soft light and the comforting smells and the familiar feelings that greet your return. Notice the light, the colors, the fragrance of your sanctuary. Notice, too, your own sense of contentedness and belonging.

"Now in your sanctuary, notice a path. You are standing, now, on the path, and you are looking off to where it stretches into the distance. You begin

to step along the path, and as you do so, you see in the distance that a form is moving towards you, radiating a clear, bright light. As you and the form of the other person approach one another, you begin to see who it is; you notice how they look and how they are dressed. The closer the person gets to where you are the more details you see in their face and their appearance.

"Gently, greet them. You are aware now that the face that is looking at you is full of wisdom and love; the eyes shine with recognition and love; this wisdom and love are just for you now. This person knows you well. They have an important and helpful message to give you, a message to guide you in your present life. You may know exactly what the message relates to, but you may be confused and not understand right now. Wordlessly, they gaze directly into your eyes, communicating this special message.

"Listen carefully to what they are saying. Listen to what they have to teach. Welcome the advice they have for you. Ask questions if you wish. You may receive the answer now – but if not, don't be discouraged; the answers will come to you soon.

"Before your visit ends, you will notice that your guide has a gift for you. This has been specially chosen to help you at this moment in your own journey. Reach out and welcome this thoughtful gift. This gift will help you on your journey towards healing.

"When the experience of being together feels complete for now, thank your guide, express your appreciation, and remind yourself that you will meet again in your sanctuary. This place and your guide are with you always. The light surrounding your guide encompasses you both.

"Calmly, and when you are ready, turn slowly back onto the path, and begin to move into the present. Begin to pay attention to your breathing. Begin to come gently awake into your body, aware of your weight on the chair. Slowly begin to shift about, moving your hands and feet. Smiling, eyes soft, gently begin to open your eyes.

"Look around. Rejoin our group. Your body is rested, awake, aware, and ready."

SUMMARY

Grief is a process of change or transition away from the immediate crisis of loss and suffering. In this time of change or transition we move slowly towards learning to live with the bonds of love and attachment without being caught in the bondage of suffering. It is a long, slow, time-consuming, and painful healing process, a journey towards human wholeness.

Grieving is never really finished. We will have "unfinished grief" right up until the moment of our own death, the time when we have to let go of all that we believe is important to us. The grieving process is not a journey that can be mapped out with straight lines. We wander back and forth in the territory of grief, first holding on to and then letting go of the pain and suffering we feel.

The trapeze artist can be a symbol for grief work. Like the trapeze artist, we swing back and forth in our grief work by holding on to the memories and the legacy of goodness passed on to us – the bonds of love and connection – and letting go of whatever creates bondage and keeps us from moving on – guilt, resentment, bitterness, or the inability to forgive ourselves or others. Keep in mind that we are what connects the past to the future. Like the trapeze artist, we let go of one swing, having faith that we will find and grasp the next swing that will bring us into a whole new experience. Trapezing is an art; it takes practice to find our own natural rhythms, and to gain the confidence to let go of one swing and take the bold new action of reaching for the next swing at precisely the right moment.

Learning the art of letting go while holding on is a lifetime process. Be gentle with yourself and members of your group, because you will each be at different stages in the grief process. You may at times feel as if you and your group members need to move on and "get back to normal." It is important to realize that you and your group *are* getting on with life and that the "old normal" is gone forever. You are in a time of transition. It is a gradual building towards a new normal.

You and other members may at times feel empty. Do not rush to fill up the emptiness. This is the neutral zone – a time of waiting. This time is similar to the changes of seasons; like autumn when the leaves are gone and there seems to be a silence all around. A waiting period comes, and it is a time to rest before new life and new energy appear.

POEMS OF REMEMBRANCE

"Miss Me but Let Me Go"

When I come to the end of the road
And the sun has set for me,
I want no rites in a gloom-filled room
Why cry for a soul set free?
Miss me a little but not too long
And now with your head bowed low,
Remember the love that we once shared
Miss me – but let me go.
For this is a journey we all must take
And each must go alone.
It's all part of the Master's Plan
A step on the road to home.
When you are lonely and sick of heart
Go to friends we know,
And bury your sorrow in doing good deeds
Miss me – but let me go.

Author Unknown

"Eulogy Delivered by Neil at Nina's Bedside"
As we walk through life's forest searching for a path
and sunlight laces the leaves,
we'll know you are there.
As we climb our hills, and our breath becomes laboured,
a breeze will cool our brow and
we'll know you are there.
As we climb above the clouds of a troubled sky
into the clear blue beyond,
we'll know you are there.
And at sunset when we see a sky bruised
with the sun's struggle to stay aloft,
we will know you are there.

Nina Tymoszewicz Docherty
died April 7, 1993, aged 39.
Mother of Bruce and Liam
Wife of Neil
Friend to Sarah, Salah, and many.

"If I Had My Life to Live Over"

I'd dare to make more mistakes next time. I'd relax, I would limber up. I would be sillier than I have been this trip. I would take fewer things seriously. I would take more chances. I would climb more mountains and swim more rivers. I would eat more ice cream and less beans. I would perhaps have more actual troubles, but I'd have fewer imaginary ones.

You see, I'm one of those people who live sensibly and sanely hour after hour, day after day. Oh, I've had my moments, and if I had it to do over again, I'd have more of them. In fact, I'd try to have nothing else. Just moments, one after another, instead of living so many years ahead of each day. I've been one of those persons who never goes anywhere without a thermometer, a hot water bottle, a raincoat, and a parachute. If I had to do it again, I would travel lighter than I have.

If I had my life to live over, I would start barefoot earlier in the spring and stay that way later in the fall. I would go to more dances. I would ride more merry-go-rounds. I would pick more daisies.

Nadine Stair

CANCER SELF-HELP GROUPS

Using Humor

"THE NIGHTLY RITUAL"
I prop my wig on the dresser
And tuck my prosthesis beneath
And thank God, I still go to bed with
My man and my very own teeth!

Janet Henry[51]

9

I find there are many fearful things we can laugh at together once we've allowed ourselves to be truly afraid.[47]

Groups are most effective when there is mutual respect, a shared sense of purpose, tolerance for conflict, and a strong feeling of cohesiveness. Many people have also described the importance of laughter during group meetings. Laughter balances the darkness of the cancer experience, as well as providing a way for connecting with others. A good meeting is often described as one where there is a lot of laughter. The ability of group members to laugh and use humor, enhances the work of any support group.

More than thirty years ago, Norman Cousins discovered something we are just beginning to acknowledge: laughter can help us heal. In 1964, Cousins, the editor of *The Saturday Review*, was diagnosed with ankylosing spondylitis, a disease which causes the spine to degenerate. His doctors told him he had a one-in-five-hundred chance of surviving. He took charge of his own treatment – and made sure it included laughter. The whole time he was sick he watched old Marx Brothers' movies, read jokes, and had friends tell them to him – in the belief that the positive feelings he got while laughing could strengthen his immune system.

Not only did he recover, he found his calling. "I have learned never to underestimate the capacity of the human mind and body to regenerate, even when the prospects seem most wretched," he wrote in his groundbreaking book *Anatomy of an Illness as Perceived by a Patient*. When part of the book was published in *The New England Journal of Medicine* in 1976, it caused a sensation. As Cousins explained in his later book, *Head First: The Biology of Hope and the Healing Power of the Human Spirit*, hearty laughter is like vigorous exercise. "It causes huffing and puffing, speeds up the heart rate, raises blood pressure, increases oxygen consumption, gives the muscles of the face and stomach a workout and relaxes other muscles." He used a great phrase to describe all this. "A belly laugh is internal jogging."

There is strong physical evidence that humor can help heal. According to researchers Lee Berk and Stanley Tan at California's Loma Linda University, "Mirthful laughter induces chemical, molecular benefits throughout our whole body. When you say, 'I feel good all over' that makes a lot of sense. We are capable of influencing our biochemistry by our mood. The evidence keeps piling up; it's just that we've only just started paying attention recently." Many other cultures have long known about this. The Greeks built their healing places near their outdoor theaters, so patients could watch performances as part of their treatments. Socrates declared, "You can't heal the body without the soul."

Now that the idea of humor as healing has caught on, there are a number of ways that cancer groups have begun to spread the word to members. Humor rooms are becoming common in hospitals, and comedy carts are found in hospitals across the country. Loretta LaRoche, who lectures extensively on the curative powers of humor and has a D.M.A. ("Doesn't Mean Anything"), teaches that "life is not a dress rehearsal". LaRoche, an adjunct member of the Mind/Body Medical Institute, an affiliate of the Harvard Medical School, speaks to countless groups about using humor and reducing stress. Her videos are used in many hospitals, and she is the author of RELAX – *You May Only Have a Few Minutes Left*. "The science is all well and good," says LaRoche. "This is a society that thrives on facts. 'If we can up our killer T cells, we just might start laughing.' But you know it's just common sense that laughter works. Laughter is connected to joy, which is connected to gratefulness. Gratefulness at being alive."

In a recent study[48] of terminally ill cancer patients living in a hospice, fourteen people were questioned about the word humor and whether humor had been a part of their life before illness. Eighty-five per cent felt that humor would be helpful in their present life. Yet only 14 per cent had any humor in their life at the time of the study. Eighty-five per cent also said that humor generated hope. They said that they had gained a sense of belonging or connectedness from shared humor, and that humor helped them to change their views of otherwise overwhelming situations and enhanced their sense of joy or pleasure and physical relaxation.

HOW TO INTRODUCE HUMOR INTO CANCER GROUPS

Used appropriately, humor can be an effective way to build positive relationships between members and improve the spirit in your group. But telling jokes isn't something that everyone is confident doing. Humor can be tricky. A light touch is essential. There are thousands of ways to encourage laughter and joyful feelings. Here are a few suggestions about the use of humor:

1. One of the simplest ways to use healing laughter is through story-telling. Set the tone by modeling your ability to "tell stories on yourself" whenever appropriate. One participant told this story.

> Rose was attending a very serious medical conference. She was feeling out of place because it seemed that everyone present was a doctor using a beeper or a cell phone or a lap-top computer. Rose was "beeper-less" and feeling very unimportant. So, she went home that night, and came back the next day to the conference with a big smile on her face . . . wearing her garage-door opener.

2. Build humor into your group culture or spirit. Some hospitals now have humor carts or humor rooms with toys, games, jokes, and videos for patients and staff. Include some humorous books or joke books in your group library.

3. Remember to use humor as a tool not a weapon. Laughing *with* others builds confidence, brings people together, and pokes fun at our common dilemmas. Laughing *at* others destroys confidence, erodes teamwork, and embarrasses others. Use humor to help *build* connections in groups.

Humor should not be used when a serious conversation is taking place or as a defence against discussing difficult emotions. Humor used this way changes the subject and does not help the group. When this happens, the group needs to bring the focus back to the difficult issue.

Consider these tips from Loretta LaRoche[49]:

1. Buy something silly and wear it. A Groucho Marx mustache and glasses are my favorite. Put them on in situations where you tend to see only the worst outcome. I wear mine when I drive through Boston, especially when I have to merge. People always let me in.

2. Write down your favorite profanities and then assign each of them a number. If someone is getting on your nerves, don't curse; just say the number. They'll never know. When they walk by, say "four".

3. Be in the moment. Don't put off your happiness or your life for a better time. There's a saying that I often use to close my lectures: "Yesterday is history. Tomorrow is a mystery. And today is a gift. That's why they call it the present."

Things I learned from my dog.[50]

+ Never pass up the opportunity for a joyride.
+ When a loved one comes home, always run to greet them.
+ When it's in your best interest, practise obedience.
+ Take naps and stretch before rising.
+ Run, romp, and play daily.
+ Eat with gusto and enthusiasm.
+ Be loyal.
+ Never pretend to be something you're not.
+ If what you want lies buried, dig until you find it.
+ When someone is having a bad day, be silent, sit close, and nuzzle them.
+ Thrive on attention and let people touch you.
+ Avoid biting when a simple growl will do.
+ On hot days, drink plenty of water and lie under a shady tree.
+ When you're happy, dance around and wag your body.
+ Bond with your pack.
+ Delight in the joy of a long walk.

The Healing Journey: Using Your Mind to Foster a Healing Environment in Your Body

Dr. Alastair Cunningham,
Ph.D., C.Psych.
Senior scientist, Ontario Cancer Institute
Edited by Pat Kelly

10

Self-help groups and facilitated support groups offer many benefits to people with cancer and their families – a chance to share the emotional burden, to regain hope, to learn ways of coping from more experienced people. Groups can help us feel we are not struggling alone in a strange and fearful land. As a cancer survivor myself, and a researcher and clinical psychologist working with cancer patients for twenty years, I am a strong believer in and advocate of this kind of emotional and practical support. In this chapter, however, I want to try to add something more; to say that, once we have decided to share and let the example of others help us, we have opened the door to a tremendous potential inside ourselves. This is the potential to discover hidden abilities in our own minds which allow us to connect more deeply with our own mind and spirit. Learning and exercising psychological and spiritual skills can make a world of difference to the experience of having cancer.

These skills can also help us to die peacefully, if that is to happen. In many cases, cancer patients who have practised these skills have lived longer, sometimes much longer, than was expected.

These may sound like large claims; they are based on research results from around the world that I will refer to later in this chapter. Researchers in the new field of psycho-oncology – meaning the study of interactions between mind and cancer – have been at great pains to prove something that is obvious to anyone with experience in an effective support group, namely, that this kind of support improves quality of life. Yet the vast majority of cancer patients do not yet receive this kind of help, and it is not part of regular cancer management.

Research has moved even farther beyond current medical practice, however, in demonstrating two additional important things about psychological self-help: first, if we add training in specific coping skills to support, cancer patients' quality of life improves even more (about twice as much as with support alone); second, and more controversially, getting keenly involved in this kind of work, undertaking what I call a "healing journey," may itself prolong life. Let's look at this further.

TWO DECISIONS FOR PEOPLE WITH CANCER

One of the first things I suggest to patients who come to our Healing Journey program is that when we are diagnosed with cancer we are faced with two major decisions. The first is: Will I be active or passive? Being passive means just presenting oneself at the clinic for medical treatment, and then trying to forget about the cancer at other times. It is the normal response in our culture, one that is often encouraged by medical centers. Becoming active, on the other hand, means looking around for ways to help oneself in addition to medical treatment.

This brings us to the second decision: What are these other "ways to heal" and where will I look for this help, "inside" myself or "outside"? "Outside" means seeking alternative remedies and procedures, things like special diets or additives or injectable substances, things that may inspire some hope and sense of control but have not yet scientifically demonstrated any effectiveness. Looking "inside" is quite different; it means exploring the potential of your own mind and spirit to help yourself. That is the approach I am advocating here. The first step in doing this is to learn some basic coping skills.

LEARNING COPING SKILLS – RELAXATION

The most basic of these skills, something that everyone could learn at school because it is so easy and effective, is deep relaxation. This is not relaxation with a glass of wine and the television, but a different kind, involving scanning the whole body for tension, and "letting it go" wherever you find it. It is a skill that needs a little practice – I would say it's about equivalent in difficulty to learning to ride a bike – but once learned, is immensely useful for counteracting stress (such as for helping you get back to sleep at those times when you wake at 3:00 a.m. with your mind whirling, or when you are sitting in the cancer clinic waiting room, or waiting by the phone, wondering what your test results will be). There are many relaxation tapes available these days (at "New Age" bookstores, for example). I suggest that you look for one that helps you to take active steps to gain intentional control over what is happening in your body, rather than just listening passively to music or a voice.

COPING SKILLS: THOUGHT WATCHING, MENTAL IMAGERY, AND GOAL SETTING

There are three or four basic coping skills to be learned. Everything else is a deepening or intensification of these basic skills. In our program, after relaxation we next introduce the idea that we can "watch" or monitor what is happening in our own minds, our own thoughts. We all have some skill at this, but we can learn to become more aware or "catch" what we are telling ourselves all the time. It is a very important skill, because our thoughts create our experience. For example, many people with cancer tell themselves constantly that their cancer is an uncontrollable disaster, that they are doomed and it's no use doing anything. The story they are telling themselves becomes their mental "world," so to speak. Our emotions closely follow our thoughts, and constant gloomy self-talk will create a depressed state. By learning to "catch" our thoughts, we can intercept such harmful patterns and either drop them or change them in a more positive direction (for example, "This pain means my body is fighting the cancer").

Better communication with others also depends on finding and acknowledging what we are truly thinking and feeling, then sharing this with someone else who is willing to listen. This kind of listening and sharing often happens very effectively in a support group.

Mental imaging means creating "pictures" (or impressions of sounds or touch or other sensations) in our minds. When we imagine something vividly, our bodies don't know the difference between the mental picture and the "real thing," and we respond as if the imagined thought is real. This is something that professional athletes, people in business, actors, and others have understood for a long time, but it has not yet been accepted into regular health-care practices.

Mental imagery has many uses in healing; at the simplest level it can be used to relax. (Imagine being on holiday or with people you love and care for. Your body will respond accordingly!) It is a way of defusing anxiety. For example, when I went into the operating room for cancer surgery, not knowing what might be found, I surrounded myself and the surgical team with a cocoon of light, and I was then able to face it all peacefully. Many patients have told me similar stories. There has been a lot written over the last few decades about imagining our body's defence systems attacking or overcoming cancer. This is a control strategy that many patients find helpful.

We don't yet have the research to document whether it has any of the hoped-for effects. Imagery can be used also to "contact" a spiritual figure, such as God or Jesus or the Buddha, or to get in touch with our inner (that is, unconscious) wisdom by invoking an "Inner Healer" with whom we can converse. Imagery has been used by some to explore facets of themselves, personified as inner characters, and to help these symbolic figures grow and mature, with apparent healing consequences. Imagery is not a trick or device; it is, rather, a language, and an immensely powerful one. Unfortunately, it still tends to be undervalued in our materialistic world.

Setting goals is also important, because without a compelling reason to live, neither our minds nor our bodies are likely to make the best possible effort to resist a life-threatening disease. We can use relaxation, followed by mental imagery, to get a mental picture of what we truly value. In one of our class exercises we ask people to picture in their imagination an ideal day, some years in the future, to see themselves as healthy and doing whatever would be most meaningful for them. After "coming back" from the relaxed state they then write a paragraph or two in order to affirm and preserve what has been learned.

These, then, are the basic, psychological self-help techniques. Many people learn much of this by themselves, using books and tapes, although it is usually easier if you have an experienced teacher. A self-help group can help its members by finding experienced and credible teachers whose task is to explain and conduct people through the techniques described; this can be a valuable addition to self-help, just as providing information about cancer and its medical treatments also helps. Our research shows that almost anyone can learn and apply these methods, but only a tiny proportion of cancer patients do so. Why? I think because this approach is unfamiliar, even scary, to many, and because it is not advocated as a part of regular treatment. It also requires a bit of effort, about half an hour to an hour of daily practice. But the effects – relief of anxiety and depression – are abundantly worth it. Other benefits include relief of physical symptoms such as fatigue, tension, and pain, plus gaining a sense of personal control that counteracts the "victim" mentality that people with cancer can experience.

MORE ADVANCED "COPING"

The kinds of self-help work described here are part of a process, one that doesn't happen all at once. That is why I call it a "journey." The journey can be undertaken in different ways to suit different people's styles or needs. However, to be most effective the process must be progressive, and not a "flitting about" from one enticing technique to another.

What happens after the basics? Very few health-care centers offer more advanced instruction in coping techniques tailored specifically for cancer patients. Enterprising people may be able to put together their own program by attending workshops and classes that are available to the public. In our own courses, the advanced program or "Stage II" offers a review of the early methods, taking the practices to greater depths, and introduces three main new techniques – meditation, the "Inner Healer" method for consulting unconscious wisdom, and the keeping of a psychological journal (exploring and recording the significant emotional events of each day).

Meditation, of course, is a process that has been known for centuries in most cultures. There are numerous meditation methods, but the basic aim is to achieve focused concentration in the relative absence of thought. Over and above its calming effects on the body, we find in meditation that we make contact with aspects of ourselves beyond the usual limited awareness of thoughts and sensations. Thus we may gain insights into our "deeper" mind, answers to troubling questions, and an understanding of what is important to us that has not come in the usual state of "busy" consciousness. But most of all, meditation is a route to contacting (becoming aware of) a higher or transcendent order or power or intelligence that has been given many names throughout history: God, the One, the Tao, the Universal Mind, and so on. The "spiritual path" is pursuing this awareness and under-standing through meditation, reflection, and harmonious action. When we are seeking to heal ourselves, this work often brings a sense of meaning to otherwise inexplicable events in life, including cancer. Self-healing techniques such as the ones described here can provide comfort and support, leading to active acceptance of whatever happens to us (which does not at all mean giving up). The person who learns coping skills and meditation and spirituality inevitably comes face to face with a search for meaning, and finds that the question "Why did this happen to me?" is closely bound to such questions as "What is the meaning of my life? What am I meant to do with my life?" As many have found – among them the wonderful people with cancer with whom I have been privileged to work – answers to these fundamental issues can be learned through the spiritual journey. Resolving these questions has brought peace for many.

If these ideas are new to you they may not make sense at first. But if you really want to help yourself, please keep an open mind and explore further. How can you do this? You may want to find a group that is already learning and practising self-healing techniques. Or perhaps you could discuss how your group members might learn more about the techniques described. You will need a trained leader who can help you understand how your mind functions, with a view to learning new and helpful practices (and unlearning old and harmful

CANCER SELF-HELP GROUPS

ones). This psychological work may be difficult and may go on for a long time, but it is most rewarding. It clears the way for the ultimate phase, the spiritual search and discovery of meaning. You will likely need a qualified teacher for this also. He or she might well be a meditation teacher or leader in some established spiritual discipline, which might be any one of many schools, including yoga, Buddhism, or a Christian or Jewish spiritual discipline. Make sure you choose a teacher who lives his or her own teachings!

WHAT EFFECTS MIGHT A HEALING JOURNEY HAVE ON PROGRESSION OF CANCER?

Research here is at an early stage. You may have heard of the widely publicized experiment of Irvine Yalom, David Spiegel, and others at Stanford University. They provided up to one year of supportive group therapy to women with metastatic breast cancer. Other women with similar disease who were randomly selected did not receive the group support. Ten years later, those who had been in the groups were found to have lived, on average, twice as long as those who had not had this kind of help. This experiment has naturally generated a lot of interest among those advocating psychological methods as an adjunct to cancer treatment. It was followed by a similar study in people with malignant melanoma (skin cancer) which also seemed to suggest that psychological self-help could prolong life. However, there are some puzzling features in the Spiegel study, notably a pattern of unusually early deaths among the women who did not get group support. The melanoma results have also not, apparently, held up after ten years.

Our own group has recently concluded a study very similar to Spiegel's in which we did not find a significant increase in average survival in women receiving group support. What does this mean? One conclusion is that we will need a larger number of experiments like these, where a group getting psychological help is compared with another that does not get the same help, before we can say whether or not this prolongs life. However, there is another way to approach the problem. Instead of looking at the average survival of groups of people, we can follow individuals closely over a number of years, as they battle their cancer, and see if different kinds of psychological adaptation are related to living longer or shorter times. We have recently completed the first (five-year) study of this kind, and the patterns are clear: in a sample of twenty-two patients with medically incurable metastatic disease who came to a support and therapy group for up to one year, those patients who became strongly involved with their psychological self-help invariably lived more than twice as long as predicted (by a panel of oncologists), and two of them have had complete, long-lasting remissions of disease! By contrast, those who did not do much of this kind of work, although no more ill, initially, than the keen individuals, did not as a rule outlive their predicted lifespan to the same extent (nearly everyone in the group did better than expected to some degree).

How could this work, physiologically? How could an intangible thing like mind affect a concrete thing like a tumor? In spite of decades of laboratory research, we know surprisingly little about the way the body controls cancers, although we do know that there are regulatory mechanisms, such as the immune system, and we understand now that cancer is not simply an "invasion" by a completely independent group of tumorous cells, but represents also a failure of these regulators to control potentially dangerous cells that are arising all the time. The mind, which we can think of as the "software" operating or emerging from the brain, has a very potent role in regulating most functions in the body – just think of the different states your body gets into when you have had a severe shock, as opposed to when you feel excited by a new project or a piece of unexpected good news. We now know that the mind strongly influences the immune system. So, although we cannot spell out in detail how the mind might assist the body to control cancer, it is evident that the mind can be the agency through which we attempt to restore balance and harmony in all aspects of our lives, with the conviction that this harmony will be translated into optimal balance in the body, the best possible state for healing. This is, of course, a very old idea, but one which we have tended to undervalue in the modern era, preferring to rely on drugs to reverse the effects of poor lifestyle and thoughtstyle.

The type of experiment I've described above, in which we follow individuals in detail, is less convincing to medical scientists than the "randomized trials," in which some people get help and others don't. It is, however, more humane (nobody is refused help) and teaches us much more about what individuals who get good medical results actually do. So we are pursuing this line of investigation; it is early yet, and there is little financial support available. However, if you have cancer, whether at a primary or a metastatic stage, I strongly recommend that you become involved with your own healing journey. Even if you feel that "the doctor got it all," your own efforts to provide optimal balance and harmony in your life and in your body may well make recurrence less likely. My enthusiasm for this course of action is based not only on the results of these formal experiments, but also on close observation of hundreds of patients over the years, and on my own experience in helping myself against cancer. At the very least, it will ease the experience for you. At best, it may prolong or save your life.

Using the Internet for Information, Support, and Advocacy

Dr. Juanne Nancarrow Clarke

11

There are thousands of sites which mention cancer on the Internet. One day, and on a casual basis, we counted the number of breast-cancer hits alone and found over 30,000. The number of hits may make the prospect of using the Internet for yourself or your group a daunting one. With a little help, though, the Internet can become an incredibly rich resource. There are sites that provide information about the latest research results, those that include calls for patients to become involved in new experimental treatments, commercial sites offering services, and alternative and complementary health-care information, among other things. There are also sites through which you can give and receive immediate interaction for support. These are real-time chat rooms, listservers, and newsgroups.

Research about on-line social and emotional support has discovered that people talk about the same things they do in "real" support groups and that many people feel that they develop a sense of "community" that is every bit as powerful as any in a real-life community. The example springs to mind of a man who, within hours of the death of his thirty-three-year-old wife, logged on to her support group to tell them of her death and to thank them for the support that she had received from the group during her illness and last days. This story points to one of the potential benefits of on-line support. If a person is unable to leave the house, or for some reason or other cannot or won't meet with others "locally," he or she is able to have ongoing, daily (or more frequent) interaction with others in similar circumstances.

For example, one woman, whose husband was living with colon cancer, was reassured to learn that many cancer patients who are unable to sleep find comfort on the Internet through late-night chat rooms for survivors. It was a relief to know that her husband wasn't alone and worrying all night about his illness.

Support groups offered on line have even been found to have an advantage over "real-life" support groups in some ways. People who want to remain anonymous can do so and still experience the benefits of the on-line groups. The Internet allows people who are geographically distant from a support group, but who have access to a computer, to participate. Because on-line support is potentially available twenty-four hours a day, people do not have to be alone in a crisis while they wait for the next meeting. It is possible to be as inactive or active as one wants to be, as there is neither a group leader asking for comments, nor peer pressure "expecting" participation.

There is a growing body of research on the particular benefits of on-line support for people with AIDS, various types of cancers, new mothers with alcohol and drug addictions, and caregivers of others (such as those with Alzheimer's).

The effectiveness of the Internet for advocacy/networking with people who have cancer has yet to be determined, but research on other issues has demonstrated the particular and powerful benefits of on-line organizing among geographically dispersed people who share a common interest. There are several instances of successful Internet organizing activities among Aboriginal communities, for instance.

In spite of the tremendous value of the Internet, it presents considerable difficulties for two main reasons – its overwhelming size and its lack of standards or regulation. The overwhelming size makes the Internet similar to approaching the archives of the *New York Times* newspaper with all of the pages of all of the papers from the time of its initial circulation piled, one on top of the other, to about the height of the Empire State Building. People around the world are working on a way to provide tables of contents, indexes, and site evaluations, as well as software for people seeking self-specialized information. In the meantime, however, finding what you need on the Internet can take time!

Instead of a central cataloguing system, the World Wide Web offers a choice of dozens of different search engines, subject guides, meta-search engines, and so on. One strategy is to go to the search engine called Yahoo and log on. Click on *Diseases* under the *Health* category, then type *cancer* in the box and do a search. You will find about 2,000 sites organized into such categories as *Health> Diseases and Conditions> Breast Cancer* and *Full Coverage> Health> Cancer Research*. Select sites of interest and learn.

Following are web addresses of various sites:

* American Association for Cancer Research (*www.aacr.org*)
* American Cancer Society (*www.cancer.org*)
* Association of Cancer Online Resources (*www.acor.org*)
* Association of Oncology Social Work (*www.aosw.org*)
* Cancer Information Service (*cis.nci.nih.gov*)
* CancerNet (*cancernet.nci.nih.gov*)
* CancerNews on the Net (*www.cancernews.com*)
* CancerWeb (*www.infoventures.com*)
* CanSearch (*www.cansearch.org*)
* Dr. Susan Love (*www.susanlovemd.com*)
* Mayo Clinic Cancer Resource Center (*www.mayohealth.org*)
* OncoLink (*www.oncolink.upenn.edu*)
* Strength from Caring (*www.onco/ink.upenn.edu/sfc*)

Planning, Reviewing, and Evaluating with Your Group

Facilitate what is happening rather than what you think ought to be happening.

The Tao of Leadership

12

GROUP SEASONS AND CYCLES

There is cyclical, seasonal, and predictable nature to the life cycle of groups. The cycle often parallels the school year. Beginning in the fall, group members will feel a surge in energy, and their attendance will improve. This is a good time to do some planning for the year ahead. Advance planning gives the group a perspective on what they will be doing and prevents them from feeling overwhelmed when demands start adding up!

Fall is often a good time to talk about planning any special events or speakers; for example, you might want to organize special activities for Cancer Awareness Month (April), National Cancer Survivor's Day (in June), and Breast Cancer Awareness Month (October). It is also a good time for members to switch roles with other members, take on new tasks, or have a respite from responsibilities.

If your group has a budget, find out what conferences or events your members want to attend during the year and plan for these expenses. If you decide to start projects such as a newsletter or a fund-raising campaign, you will need to find volunteers and start planning early. Some groups will decide on a date for special rituals or ceremonies to remember and celebrate the lives of members.

September, January, and June are the times many groups reflect on or evaluate group meetings. Think about what is working well, and ask members if their needs and expectations are being met. Schedule a time for reviewing the role of the facilitators, and invite other group members to consider learning the skills necessary to assume this role. Plan to participate in a facilitation workshop. Experienced facilitators can plan to coach new people and mentor them until they gain the skills and confidence they need.

CANCER SELF-HELP GROUPS

EVALUATION

Several times during the year it will be helpful to take stock of what is working for your members and what isn't. In any group, things sometimes come to a standstill. Members may become bored, frustrated, lacking in energy, less committed, or interested in other issues. If members expect one thing from group and are getting something else, they may become frustrated and leave. When members are leaving and you don't know why, an evaluation can help your group understand what is happening; then discuss ways to make changes. Evaluation is a process for measuring what is working for your group and what needs changing. It is not a judgment about success or failure.

According to research, [51] effective cancer self-help groups:

+ provide members with acceptance, warmth, humor, a welcoming atmosphere, and
+ a source of energy;
+ have few rules, a clear purpose, and an agreed-upon code of behavior;
+ encourage cooperation, shared decision-making, open communication, and confidentiality.

You might ask members to discuss these characteristics and consider how your group is doing in these areas. This can help identify places that need work or where members may have skills that can be used to improve your meetings.

Some groups wait until the group is really in trouble before they sit down and try to understand what is happening. However, ongoing evaluation which is planned and a part of the normal activities for your group is one way to ensure that the group has clear goals and *evaluation*

that the goals are being achieved. Evaluation should not interfere with the group or be threatening in any way.

There are several ways to do evaluation. The group can have a candid discussion, members can be asked to fill out forms, the facilitators' journal can be a resource, or an experienced outside observer can sit in on a group meeting and describe the process as he or she sees it. One or two times a year your group should plan an evaluation time. The purpose is to find out if members receive the support, information, and guidance they expected. You can also ask members how joining the group has affected their relationships with friends, family, and doctors. The sample Evaluation of Satisfaction form on page 56 can help.

GROUP DISCUSSION

The easiest way for a group to evaluate itself is through group discussion. The process will require a group member to act as a leader or facilitator for the evaluation meeting. However, if the group members will also be commenting on the facilitation process, ask someone other than the facilitators to lead the evaluation. You will need to record the findings and recommendations – perhaps on a flip chart. This will be helpful for planning changes and as a written record of the group decision-making process.

Useful questions include:

1. What were you expecting to get when you first joined the group?
2. What is one thing you appreciate about the group?
3. How do you view your own participation?
4. How do you feel about the role you have played?
5. Describe a good experience you remember in group.
6. Describe one thing you would like to have happen in group.

7. Describe a gift or skill you bring to group.

8. Describe what you understand the purpose of the group to be.

The sample of a confidential group evaluation form shown on page 56 may help your group. Once your members have completed the evaluation process, use the findings about what is working and what needs to change and brainstorm ideas about how to make changes happen. Set out a plan and timetable and indicate who is responsible for the actions or activities. Report back to your group about the evaluation and the planning. Keep a record of the evaluation and plans in the group journal. Knowing what changes are coming up will help members to feel involved and increase their sense of belonging in the group. Keeping members informed about planned changes can help you to avoid anxiety about changes to the meeting location or schedule or about having new facilitators.

Don't be upset if, despite your best efforts, members react with surprise and confusion when they first experience something new or different. Human beings are flawed and forgetful – even the special folks who are part of your cancer group.

SUMMARY

1. In the fall, think about planning ahead for special events, speakers, and new projects.

2. About three times a year, try to review the facilitators' role.

3. Several times a year, use group discussion to evaluate what is working for your members and what isn't.

4. Sample Evaluation of Satisfaction form (page 56).

Making Connections Beyond the Group

Learn to lead in a nourishing manner.
The Tao of Leadership

13

NETWORKING WITH OTHER CANCER SELF-HELP GROUPS

Your group may want to network with other cancer self-help groups for a lot of reasons:

+ to share resources;
+ to get advice or coaching when you are getting started;
+ to build coalitions for fundraising or advocacy;
+ to attend workshops together;
+ to learn different perspectives;
+ to support one another through difficult times;
+ to build confidence;
+ to educate the public;
+ to collaborate on projects.

Even if your cancer self-help group does not want formal partnerships with other cancer groups or organizations, you will likely meet people from other groups, especially if you are doing community outreach or working on committees or boards which provide cancer-care services.

TIPS FOR NETWORKING WITH OTHER SELF-HELP GROUPS

+ Get in touch with other group facilitators and ask how you might share ideas, provide support or encouragement for each other, or work together on projects.
+ Attend each other's meetings as guests.
+ Find opportunities for joint meetings, retreats, and workshop training.

- Get together by phone or letter to give each other moral support and share skills.
- Have a joint group meeting on a common issue and invite a guest speaker.
- Start a joint newsletter.

NETWORKING WITH AGENCIES AND CANCER-CARE INSTITUTIONS

- Invite nurses, oncologists, or other cancer experts as guest speakers.
- Offer to speak at the institution about your group.
- Seek opportunities for joint workshops or advocacy efforts.
- Plan joint activities or ask them to sponsor guest speakers that interest both groups.
- Offer to write an article about your group for their newsletter.

DEVELOPING GOOD RELATIONSHIPS WITH HEALTH-CARE PROVIDERS

Whatever the nature of the partnership between self-help groups and cancer professionals, there must be mutual respect, tolerance, an understanding of each other's role, and commitment in order for any partnership to work. The members of the cancer self-help group need to be clear about what they want from the professionals they choose to work with. Groups may value professionals' participation because it may give them access to resources and expertise. Professionals may refer people to the group. Professional support can give your group more credibility, especially with policy makers and other professionals. Professionals also value self-help groups as a way of helping their patients get emotional support and practical help in dealing with their concerns.

HOT TIPS

♦ Choose professionals who share common values with your group.
♦ Learn about potential partners.
♦ Decide what the purpose and goals of the partnership will be.
♦ Follow up contacts with a call or letter.
♦ Keep a file of the contacts and information shared.
♦ Educate professionals about the benefits of cancer self-help groups.
♦ Decide what role you need the professional to play – consultant, mentor, provider of information, provider of referrals to group.
♦ Remember that professionals can play public and private roles.
♦ Evaluate your relationships and outcomes from time to time.

PROMOTING YOUR GROUP

♦ Be able to describe yourself well.
♦ Create a brochure describing your history, goals, and meetings and identifying your contact person.
♦ Advertise your group in hospitals, doctors' offices, and social workers' and counselors' offices.

DEVELOPING EFFECTIVE RELATIONSHIPS WITH THE MEDIA

Working with the media may or may not be something your group wants to do. However, cancer is a very popular topic in the media, and human-interest stories about people living with the disease are often used to explain the importance of new discoveries and treatments. You should know how your group wants to be represented in order to answer questions about it.

HOT TIPS

- Know your message. Get group consensus on how you want to describe your group, and be consistent with the messages.
- Get to know the media. Try to get to know staff from TV and radio stations, newspapers, and magazines. Set up a meeting and introduce your group.
- Have a trained, designated spokesperson.
- Target your audience. The media are not your target. You need them to reach your real audience.
- Be prepared. Use only facts that you *know* are current and reliable. When media representatives interview you about your group or issue, they assume you know what you are talking about. Do some research. Don't pretend to know something you don't. Ask if you can get back to them with an answer. Then do it.
- Make clear guidelines about confidentiality for your group.
- Stay focused and *get your message across clearly*.

SUMMARY

1. Network with other cancer self-help groups.
2. Network with health-care providers.
3. Learn how to work with the media to promote your group.

Closing

A good group is better than a spectacular group.
The Tao of Leadership

14

This guide provides an outline of what cancer self-help groups can do and some ideas about how to start and maintain effective groups. Our intention was to provide some directions and encouragement for your work. We hope we have increased your understanding of the impact of cancer and have helped you discover and plan a way for your group to work together to meet the needs of your members. We would also like to share with you some reasons why we – the author and other members of cancer groups – do this work.

Twelve years ago, when the first cancer self-help groups were getting started, self-help members were considered a small band of rebels – radicalized by our cancer. We were seeking new ways to heal and to learn to live with disease. Our goal was to look everywhere for effective ways that might help us bring meaning and vitality into our lives.

Today, there are many more "rebels and radicals" starting and leading cancer self-help groups.

Today, although we are more experienced and better trained than when we began, we are still seeking new ways of healing. We still love what we do. And we still gain tremendous satisfaction from enriching the lives of other people living with cancer.

Being involved as a member of a cancer support group can be rewarding, powerful, and challenging work. Groups can also become a source of comfort, knowledge, courage, and humor, and our lives are immeasurably enriched by group friendships.

Celebrate together – your lives and your work!

> The bottom line is that once a month I get together with a room full of
> women, all of whom have breast cancer. And just the air in the room is
> a relief to breathe.

NOTES

Introduction

1 American Cancer Society, 1999.

Chapter 1

2 Adapted with permission from David Cella and Suzanne Yellen, "Cancer Support Groups: The State of the Art," *Cancer Practice* 1, no. 1 (May/June 1993).

3 The author uses the definition of cancer survivor provided by the National Coalition for Cancer Survivorship: anyone with a history of cancer from the point of diagnosis and for the remainder of life.

4 R. Gray et al., "A Qualitative Study of Breast Cancer Self-help Groups," *Journal of Psycho-oncology*, 6 (1997): 279–89.

5 Adapted from Cella and Yellen, "Cancer Support Groups: The State of the Art."

6 Health Canada National Forum on Breast Cancer, 1993 Survey of Breast Cancer Survivors.

7 Gray et al., "A Qualitative Study of Breast Cancer Self-help Groups."

8 Adapted from Cella and Yellen, "Cancer Support Groups: The State of the Art."

9 Ibid.

10 Gray et al., "A Qualitative Study of Breast Cancer Self-help Groups."

11 Adapted from Cella and Yellen, "Cancer Support Groups: The State of the Art."

12 Ibid.

13 Gray et al., "A Qualitative Study of Breast Cancer Self-help Groups."

14 Adapted from Cella and Yellen, "Cancer Support Groups: The State of the Art."

15 L.F. Kurtz, "The Self-help Movement: Review of the Past Decade of Research," *Social Work with Groups* 13, no. 3 (1990): 101–15.

16 Cunningham, A.J., Edmonds, C.V.I., Jenkins, E.P., Pollack, H., Lockwood, G.A., and Warr, D. (1998) A randomized control trial of the effects of group psychological therapy on survival in women with metastic breast cancer. *Psycho-Oncology* 7, 508-17.

17 Adapted from Cella and Yellen, "Cancer Support Groups: The State of the Art," and from Bonnie Pope, *Self-Help/Mutual Aid*, Canadian Mental Health Association, Social Action Series, Ottawa, 1991.

18 F. Lavoie, T. Borkman, and B. Gidron, *Self-help and Mutual Aid Groups: International and Multicultural Perspective* (New York: Haworth Press, 1994).

19 Kurtz, "The Self-help Movement: Review of the Past Decade of Research." *Social Work with Groups*, 13, no. 3 (1990): 101-15.

CHAPTER 2

20 Adapted from Ram Dass and Mirabi Bush, *Compassion in Action: Setting Out on the Path of Service* (New York: Bell Tower Press, 1992).

21 Adapted from *The Self-Help Sourcebook*, 6th ed. (Danville, NJ: American Self-Help Clearinghouse, 1998).

22 Adapted from Carol Town, *Towards Effective Self-help – A Group Facilitation Training Manual* (The Prevention Network of Hamilton-Wentworth, January 1993).

23 Treya William Wilber, "What Kind of Help Really Helps?" 1988. Reprinted with permission from the Cancer Support Community, San Francisco.

CHAPTER 3

24 Bruce Tuckman, "The Stages of Group Development" in *Conducting Educational Research*, 3rd ed. (San Diego: Harcourt Brace Jovanovich, 1988).

25 Cella and Yellen

26 S.E. Taylor, R.L. Falke, S.J. Shoptaw, and R.R. Lichtman, "Social Support, Support Groups and the Cancer Patient," *Journal Consulting Clinical Psychology* (1986).

Chapter 4

27 Adapted from Cella and Yellen, "Cancer Support Groups: The State of the Art."

28 Ibid.

29 Adapted from F. Rees, *How to Lead Work Teams: Facilitation Skills* (San Diego, CA.: Pfeiffer and Company, 1991).

30 Gray et al., "A Qualitative Study of Breast Cancer Self-help Groups."

31 Wilber, "What Kind of Help Really Helps?"

32 Cella and Yellen

Chapter 6

33 Cella and Yellen

34 Wilber, "What Kind of Help Really Helps?"

35 Adapted from "Section 2: Listening Skills," ME Hotline Training Program (Chicago: Y-ME National Breast Cancer Organization, 1992).

36 Wilber, "What Kind of Help Really Helps?"

37 Ibid.

38 AIDS Committee of Toronto, *Support Group Facilitation Manual* 1996.

Chapter 7

39 Adapted from "Identifying and Handling Problem Behaviors," in American Cancer Society, *Guidelines on Support and Self-Help Groups* (American Cancer Society, Inc. 1994), Atlanta, GA, p. 63.

40 *Self-Help Leader's Handbook: Lading Effective Meetings*. Publication produced by Research and Training Center on Independent Living, University of Kansas, Lawrence, Kansas, 1991.

41 D. Murray-Ross, and C. Mederios, *Facilitation Skills Workshop*, The American Cancer Society National Conference on Support and Self-help Groups, Bellevue, WA (August 1992).

CHAPTER 8

42 Gray et al., "A Qualitative Study of Breast Cancer Self-help Groups."
44 Ibid.
45 Wilber, "What Kind of Help Really Helps?"
46 Adapted from Sandi Capelan and Gordon Lang, *Grief's Courageous Journey, A Workbook* (New Harbinger Publications: Oakland, California, 1995).

CHAPTER 9

47 Wilber, "What Kind of Help Really Helps?"
48 K. Herth, "Contributions of Humor as Perceived by the Terminally Ill," *American Journal of Hospital Care* 7, no. 1 (1990): 36–40.
49 Loretta LaRoche, *RELAX – You May Only Have a Few Minutes Left* (Random House, New York, NY: Villard, 1998).
50 Patty Wooten, *Compassionate Laughter, Jest for Your Health*, Salt Lake City, Utah: Commune-A-Key Publishing, 1996).
51 Ibid.

CHAPTER 12

51 Cella and Yellen

RESOURCES

There are resources available all across the U.S. to aid the formation of new self-help groups and to provide ideas and skills for existing groups. The resources allow groups to draw upon the wisdom gained by others. As well, the resources can provide the expertise of individuals who are dedicated to empowering the people in their community by teaching skills that are important for the success of self-help groups.

This section focuses on two aspects of making a self-help group successful. The first relates to group process skills, logistics, and administrative issues. The second relates to resources that groups can use to get ideas for discussion topics and for dealing with issues that are likely to arise.

Resources for Facilitator Training and Development

PISCES
(Partnering in Self-help Community Education and Support)

Leadership from the Heart: A two day workshop providing skills develop-

ment based upon the teachings in this manual. Led by Pat Kelly and Hugh Huntington. Programs available on site.

2021 Lakeshore Road, Suite 108
Burlington, Ontario
Canada L7R 1A2
Phone: (905) 637-2840
E-mail: *pisces@netinc.ca*
Web address: *www.pisces.on.ca*

HOLLYHOCK
Workshops—Retreats—Vacations

Training and development in a west-coast sanctuary.

Box 127, Manson's Landing
Cortez Island, British Columbia
Canada V0P 1K0
Phone: 1-800-933-6339
E-mail: *hollyhock@oberon.ark.com*
Web address: *www.hollyhock.bc.ca*

OMEGA
Institute for Holistic Studies

Training and personal development in an east-coast retreat center.

260 Lake Drive
Rhinebeck, New York

U.S.A. 12572-3212

Phone: 1-800-944-1001

Web address: *www.omega-inst.org*

Information for Self-Help Groups

There is a network of Self-Help Centers across the United States whose mandate is to provide support and consultation for new and existing self-help groups.

Services include:

♦ Directories of self-help groups
♦ Telephone information and referral
♦ Specialized workshops and training
♦ Up-to-date information on resources and research
♦ Resource library
♦ Linkages with other self-help centers

AMERICAN SELF-HELP CLEARINGHOUSE

St. Clare's Hospital

25 Pocono Road

Denville, NJ 07834

Phone: 1-800-367-6274

Web address: *www.cmhc.com/selfhelp*

Serves as a guide for exploring support groups and networks within one's community as well as internationally.

The American Self-Help Clearinghouse publishes a 344-page *Self-Help Sourcebook,*

now in its 6th edition.

SUPPORTWORKS

1018 East Boulevard

Suite 5

Charlotte, NC 28203-5779

Phone: (704) 377-2055 (Mon.-Thurs., 9 a.m.-noon)

SupportWorks publishes an excellent 8-page resource booklet called *PowerTools—Ways to Build A Self-help Group*. Bulk orders available.

SupportWorks has developed an economic telephone support group model called SupportLink. For more information about how this model can be helpful foryou, contact Joal Fisher, MD, Executive Director.

Burns, Judith and Lenko, Svetlana (with Hector Balthazar), *Resources for Self-Help* (1989). Catalogue with detailed listings of materials relating to self-care, self-help and mutual aid which are held by over 100 national volunteer organizations in Canada.

Hill, Karen (revised and updated by Hector Balthazar), *Helping You Helps Me* (1987). Still one of the most popular and useful books on self-help published in the past ten years, with over 50,000 copies sold. A practical guide to starting and maintaining a self-help group. Leadership, membership, recruitment, fund-raising, problem-solving, and decision-making are discussed among the more than twenty subjects covered.

Romeder, Jean-Marie, *The Self-Help Way: Mutual Aid and Health* (1990). This book provides a comprehensive look at the remarkable growth and development of self-help groups and the vital role they play in the lives of an increasing number of people. It probes into the dynamics of "the self-help way" which fosters equality, mutual respect, support and understanding. This work makes an important contribution to understanding the important role of self-help groups in our society.

BOOKS ABOUT SELF-HELP GROUPS

Community libraries have many books about developing successful self-help groups. Some good resource books include:

Davis Kasl, Charlotte, *Many Roads, One Journey: Moving Beyond the 12 Step Process* (1992) and *Yes You Can: A Guide to Empowerment Groups* (1995).

Sher, B., *Teamworks!: Building support groups that guarantee success* (New York: Warner Books, 1989). Readable and practical.

Silverman, P., *Mutual Help Groups: Organization and Development* (Beverly Hills: Sage Publications, 1980).

Steinberg, D.M., *The Mutual-Aid Approach to Working with Groups* (Northvale, NJ: Jason Aronson, Inc., 1998). Discusses the behaviors which make groups work, their stages of development, and strategies to deal with generic issues which often arise in groups.

HUMOR RESOURCES

Books

Adams, Patch (with Maureen Mylander), *Gesundheit! Bringing Good Health to You, the Medical System and Society Through Physician Service, Complementary Therapies, Humor and Joy* (Healing Arts Press, 1996).

Clifford, C., *Not Now ... I'm having a no hair day: Humor and Healing for people with Cancer* (Duluth, MN: Pfeifer-Hamilton, 1996), c/o: The Cancer Club, 6533 Limerick Dr, Edina, MN 55439 ($12).

Cousins, Norman, *Anatomy of An Illness*

as Perceived by the Patient (W.W. Norton, 1979).

Cousins, Norman, *Head First: The Biology of Hope and the Healing Power of the Human Spirit* (Penguin, 1989).

Klein, Allen, *The Healing Power of Humor: Techniques for Getting Through Loss, Setbacks, Upsets, Disappointments, Difficulties, Trials, Tribulations, and All That Not-so-funny Stuff* (Jeremy P. Tarcher, 1989).

LaRoche, Loretta, *RELAX—You May Only Have a Few Minutes Left: Using the Power of Humor to Overcome Stress in Your Life and Your Work* (Villard, 1998).

Wooten, Patty, *Compassionate Laughter: Jest for Your Health* (Commune-A-Key Publishing, 1996).

Organizations
American Association of Therapeutic Humor (AATH)
222 S. Meramec, Suite 303
St. Louis MO 63105
Phone: (314) 863-6232
Web address: *www.aath.org*

The Humor Project
110 Spring St.
Saratoga Springs, NY 12866
Phone: (518) 587-8770

GENERAL READING LIST

Altman, R., and Sarg, M.J., *The Cancer Dictionary* (New York, 1992).

American Cancer Information Service. *What Are Clinical Trials All About?* A 22-page booklet.

Frank, Arthur, *At the Will of the Body: Reflections on Illness* (Boston: Houghton Mifflin Co., 1991).

Frank, Arthur, *The Wounded Storyteller: Body, Illness and Ethics* (The University of Chicago Press, 1995).

Johnson, J., and Klein, L., *I Can Cope: Staying Healthy with Cancer* (Wayzata, MN: DCI Publishing, 1994).

LeShan, L., *Cancer As A Turning Point* (NY: EP Dutton, 1989).

Love, S., *Dr. Susan Love's Breast Book* (NY: Addison Wesley Longman, 1995).

Murphy, G.P., Morris, L.B., and Lange, D., *The American Cancer Society's Informed Decisions: The Complete Book of Cancer Diagnosis, Treatment and Recovery* (New York: Viking Penguin, 1997).

Nancarrow Clarke, Juanne, and Nancarrow Clarke, Lauren, *Finding Strength: A mother and daughter's story of childhood cancer* (Toronto: Oxford University Press, 1999).

Topf, L., *You Are Not Your Illness* (Toronto: Fireside, 1995).

ADVOCACY

Stabiner, K., *To Dance With The Devil: The New War on Cancer Politics, Power and People* (NY: Bantam Doubleday Dell, 1997).

COMPLEMENTARY APPROACHES

The Alternative Medicine Homepage. Links to many alternative and complementary therapies. www.pitt.edu/~chw/altm.html

Lerner, M. *Choices in Healing: Integrating the Best of Conventional and Complementary Approaches to Cancer.* Cambridge: MIT Press, 1994.

Moss, R. *Cancer Therapy: The Independent Consumer's Guide to Non-Toxic Treatment and Prevention.* New York: Equinox Press, 1992.

CHEMOTHERAPY

Bruning, N. *Coping with Chemotherapy.* New York: Ballantine Books, 1993.

Dodd, M.J. *Managing the Side Effects of Chemotherapy and Radiation Therapy: A Guide for Patients and Their Families.* San Francisco: UCSF Nursing Press, 1996.

DIET

Nixon, D.W. *The Cancer Recovery Eating Plan: The Right Foods to Help Fuel Your Recovery.* New York: Random House, 1996.

Spears, R. *Low Fat and Loving It.* New York: Warner Books, 1990.

ISSUES FOR CHILDREN WHEN A PARENT HAS CANCER

Harpham, W.S., *When a Parent Has Cancer: A Guide to Caring for Your Children with Becky and the Worry Cup* (HarperCollins, 1997).

McCue, K., *How to Help Children Through a Parent's Serious Illness* (NY: St. Martin's Press, 1994).

Video: *Kids Tell Kids What It's Like—when a family member has cancer;* Cancervive. To order call (310) 203-9232.

SUPPORT FOR CARE GIVERS

Berry, C.R., *When Helping You is Hurting Me* (NY: Harper & Row, 1989).

Das, Ram, and Gorman, P., *How Can I Help?* (NY: Knopf, 1994).

Wilson Schaef, A., *Meditations for Women Who Do Too Much* (NY: Harper and Row, 1992).

RELAXATION, MEDITATION AND VISUALIZATION RESOURCES

Achterberg, J., *Rituals of Healing: Imagery for Health and Well-being* (Bantam Books, 1994).

Bedard, Jim, *Lotus in the Fire, The Healing Power of Zen* (Shambhala, 1999).

Benson, H., *The Relaxation Response* (Avon Books, 1975).

Cunningham, A.J., *The Healing Journey: Overcoming the Crisis of Cancer* (Key Porter Books, 1999).

Epstein, G., *Healing Visualizations* (Bantam Books, 1989).

Fanning, P., *Visualization for Change* (New Harbinger, 1988).

Harpham, W., *After Cancer: A Guide to Your New Life* (Harper Perennial, 1994).

Kabat-Zinn, J., *Full Catastrophe Living* (NY: Dell Publishing, 1990).

Napanstek, B., *Staying Well with Guided Imagery* (NY: Warner Books, 1994).

CANCER ORGANIZATIONS:

American Cancer Society
1599 Clifton Road, NE
Atlanta, GA 30329
Phone: 1-800-ACS-2345
Web address: *www.cancer.org*

The ACS is a national organization with local offices throughout the U.S. It provides information and referrals to numerous local and community support services as well as maintaining a library of cancer education publications available to the public.

AMC Cancer Research Center
1600 Pier Street
Denver, CO 80214
Phone: 1-800-525-3777
Web address: *www.amc.org*

Provides information on symptoms, diagnosis, treatment, psychosocial issues, support groups, and other valuable resources, such as financial aid and transportation services.

American Self-Help Clearinghouse
St. Clare's Hospital

25 Pocono Road
Denville, NJ 07834
Phone: 1-800-367-6274
Web address: *Mentalhelp.net/selfhelp*

Serves as a guide for exploring support groups and networks within one's community as well as throughout the world.

CancerCare
275 7th Avenue
New York, NY 10001
Phone: 1-800-813-HOPE
Web address: *www.cancercare.org*

A non-profit organization providing emotional support, information and practical help to people with cancer and their families and friends. *Helping Hands: The Resource Guide for People with Cancer* is available at no extra charge.

Cancer Information Service
National Cancer Institute (NCI)
Office of Cancer Communications
31 Center Dr. MSC 2580
Bldg. 31, Room 10A16
Bethesda, MD 20892-2580
Phone: 1-800-4-CANCER
Web address: *www.nci.nih.gov*

The Cancer Information Service provides up-to-date information on cancer to patients and their families, health professionals, and the general public. Materials can be accessed on the web site or by calling CIS.

Intercultural Cancer Council
PMB—C
1720 Dryden
Houston, TX 77030
Phone: (713) 798-4617
Web address: *icc.bcm.tmc.edu*

The Intercultural Cancer Council has developed policies and programs that address the high incidence rates of cancer among minority populations.

Mautner Project for Lesbians with Cancer
1707 L. St. NW, Suite 500
Washington, DC 20036
Phone: (202) 332-5536
Web address: *www.mautnerproject.org*

This initiative offers education, information, support, advocacy and direct services for Lesbians with cancer and their loved ones.

National Asian Women's Health Organization (NAWHO)
250 Montgomery St., Ste. 410
San Francisco, CA 94104
Phone: (415) 989-9747
Web address: *www.nawho.org*

NAWHO, a non-profit agency, is a community-based health advocacy organization committed to improving the overall health status of Asian women and girls.

National Comprehensive Cancer Network
50 Huntingdon Pike, Ste. 200
Rockledge, PA 19046
Phone: 1-888-909-NCCN
Web address: *www.nccn.org*

A non-profit organization which provides reliable, specific and easy-to-understand information for cancer patients, including *Standards of Care and Treatment Guidelines for Distress Management in Cancer Survivors.*

National Health Information Center
P.O. Box 1133
Washington, DC 20013-1133
Phone: 1-800-336-4797
Web address: *www.nhic-nt.health.org*

This U.S. government agency aids consumers in locating health information.

National Women's Health Network
510 10th Street NW, Ste. 400
Washington, DC 20004
Phone: (202) 347-1140
Web address:
www.womenshealthnetwork.org

This organization provides newsletters and position papers on women's health issues and concerns.

Native C.I.R.C.L.E.
The American Indian/Alaska Native Cancer Information Resource Center and Learning Exchange
Norwest Building, Ste. 521
200 1st Street SW
Rochester, MN 55905
Phone: (877) 372-1617
Web address:
www.mayo.edu/nativecircle

Resource center for providing American Indian and Alaskan Native cancer-related materials to health-care professionals and the general public.

OMH: The Office of Minority Health
OMP P.O. Box 37337
Washington, DC 20013-7337
Phone: 1-800-444-6472
(9 a.m. to 5 p.m. EST)
Web address: *www.omhrc.gov*

The OMH maintains comprehensive databases on minority health issues and resources. Several OMH publications are available free.

Breast Cancer Organizations:

NABCO: National Alliance of Breast Cancer Organizations
9 E 37th Street, 10th Floor
New York, NY 10016
Phone: (212) 719-0154
Phone: 1-800-719-9154
Web address: *www.nabco.org*

NABCO is a non-profit resource that provides up-to-date, accurate information for patients and their families, media, professionals, and medical organizations. It provides a large variety of professionally prepared information resources.

National Breast Cancer Coalition
1707 L Street NW, Ste. 1060
Washington, DC 20036
Phone: 1-800-422-6237
Web address: *www.natlbcc.org*

The coalition advocates increased funding for breast cancer research, improved access to high-quality breast cancer screening, diagnosis, and treatment, particularly for underserved and under-insured women.

SHARE, Self-help for Women with Breast or Ovarian Cancer
1501 Broadway, Ste. 1720
New York, NY 10036

Phone: (212) 382-2111 (English)
Phone: (212) 719-4454 (Spanish)
Web address: *www.sharecancersupport.org*

A self-help organization that serves individuals affected by breast or ovarian cancer. SHARE offers English and Spanish hotlines, peer-led support groups, public education, advocacy, and wellness programs.

Sisters Network
8787 Woodway Drive, Ste. 4206
Houston, TX 77063
Phone: (713) 781-0255
Web address: *www.sistersnetworkinc.org*

An African American breast cancer survivor's organization involved in emotional support, research, cancer prevention programs and advocacy efforts.

The Susan G. Komen Breast Cancer Foundation
5005 LBJ Freeway, Suite 370
Dallas, TX 75244
Phone: 1-800-I'M-AWARE
(1-800-462-9273) (9 a.m. to 4:30 p.m. CST, Monday through Friday)
Phone: 972-855-1600
Web address: *www.komen.org*
Web address: *www.breastcancerinfo.com*
Web address: *www.raceforthecure.com*

The Komen Foundation is an international organization with a network of volunteers working through Affiliates and the Komen Race For The Cure events across the country, fighting to eradicate breast cancer as a life-threatening disease. The Foundation and its Affiliates fund research, innovative breast cancer education, screening, and treatment projects for the medically underserved in communities across the country. The Helpline (1-800-I'M-AWARE), which is answered by volunteers, provides the latest breast health information. Se habla espanol. TDD is also available.

Y-ME National Breast Cancer Organization
212 West Van Buren St., 4th Floor
Chicago, IL 60607
Phone: 1-800-221-2141 (English)
Phone: 1-800-986-9505 (Spanish)
Web address: *www.y-me.org*

Y-ME provides peer support and information to women and men who have or suspect they have breast cancer.

YWCA Encore Plus program
1025 Connecticut Ave. Ste. 1012
Washington, DC 20036
Phone: 1-800-992-2871
Web address: *www.ywca.org*

Encore Plus is a breast and cervical cancer outreach and screening program for women over 50.

ON-LINE INTERNET RESOURCES:

OncoLink—University of Pennsylvania Cancer Center
3451 Walnut
Philadelphia, PA 19104
Web address: *www.oncolink.upenn.edu*

A leading information website developed and regularly updated by the University of Pennsylvania Medical Center Staff. The site has an extensive section on psychosocial support. Other sections include art, literature, video, poetry, performing arts, cancer and sexuality, coping, and spirituality.

Computer Bulletin Boards and Listservers.
America Online (888) 265-4357, CompuServe (800) 848-8199, and prodigy (800) 776-3449, all have bulletin boards where cancer survivors exchange support and information. E-mail users can subscribe to electronic support groups and mailing lists where cancer survivors, family, friends, and health professionals share information and support through e-mail. For more information see www.acor.org/index.html.

Journal Searches.
Medline is the largest Online data-

base, with 3600 contributing journals. Medline has a separate database called Cancerlit. Some public libraries subscribe to these and will allow you to access them for a fee. Medline is available at no cost on the web through Healthcare at www.healthgate.com.

Can Search—National Coalition for Cancer Survivorship—*www.cansearch.org.*

American Association for Cancer Research—*www.aacr.org*

American Cancer Society—*www.cancer.org*

Association of Cancer Online Resources—*www.acor.org*

Association of Oncology Social Work—*www.aosw.org*

CancerNet—*cancernet.nci.nih.gov*

CancerNews on the Net—*www.cancernews.com*

CanSearch—*www.cansearch.org*

CancerWeb—*www.infoventures.com*

Cancer Information Service—*cis.nci.nih.gov*

Dr. Susan Love—*www.susanlovemd.com*

Mayo Clinic Cancer Resource Center—*www.mayohealth.org*

National Cancer Institute cancer

trials—*www.cancertrials.nci.nih.gov.*

The National Cancer Institute—*www.cancernet.nci.nih.gov.*

OncoLink—*www.oncolink.upenn.edu*

Strength from Caring—*www.oncolink.upenn.edu/sfc*

INDEX

A

achievement, 95
active involvement, 20-21, 129, 136
advocacy, 173
affirmations, 112
agreement, 58-59, 71, 101
alternative remedies and procedures, 129, 171
Anatomy of an Illness as Perceived by a Patient, 122
anonymity, 60, 141
assertive caring, 100-101
attendance, 74

B

basic principles, 30
bereavement counseling, 108
Berk, Lee, 123
Breast Cancer Awareness Month, 144
Breast Cancer Care Petition, 142
Breast Cancer Links: A Cancer News Service, 142
bridging, 89-90
budget, 144
burnout, 102-104

C

Cancer Awareness Month, 144
Cancer Support Community, 22-23
caregivers, 66, 172
ceremonies, 112-113
characteristics of self-help groups, 15, 16, 20-21, 145
chemotherapy, 171
childcare, 46,73

clinical depression, 17, 99
closed groups, 53-54
closed-ended questions, 89
CNN Health – Women's Health, 142
co-facilitators, 53, 78, 79-80
coaching, 103
code of behavior, 58-59, 71, 145
comedy carts, 123
common bonds, 18, 50-51
community meeting, 65-66
confidentiality, 60
conflicts, 46
consensus, 92
constructive action, 98
content, 83-84
control, 95-96
coping skills, 128
    advanced, 133-135
    goal setting, 132
    "Inner Healer" method, 133
    learning, 132-133
    meditation, 133-134
    mental imaging, 131-132
    psychological journal, 133
    relaxation, 130
    thought watching, 130-131
    courage to face fears, 106, 108
Cousins, Norman, 122
culture, 53, 66-67
cyclical nature of groups, 144

D

death, 16, 106-108
depression, 131
different stages of disease, 51-52
difficult behavior, 32, 97-100
discrimination, 13
diverse membership, 44-47
Docherty, Nina Tymoszewicz, 119